<u>Surgeon:</u>

The Man
Behind the Mask

RICHARD H. GERMAN, M.D., F.A.C.S.

First published by Dog Ear Publishing
4010 W. 86th Street, Ste H
Indianapolis, IN 46268
www.dogearpublishing.net

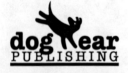

ISBN: 978-160844-465-6

This book is printed on acid-free paper.

Printed in the United States of America

READER REVIEWS

"This memoir of one surgeon's personal struggles and professional education, and early years of experience with scalpels, surgeries and sutures will reassure the reader that there is, indeed, a very human *man* behind the mask. It is an exciting and poignant insight into the very revelations involved in the life and surgical training of a young man, and the quixotic personalities that weave through the tapestry of his maturation, from med student to surgeon." —Martha Humphreys

"Dr. German's book masterfully pulls the "mask" down from the surgeon's life, thus drawing the reader into the very private world of 'medicine's back office'. German's book is as close to holding a scalpel as the reader can get . . ." –Robert Keller, M.D.

"In his book, *"Surgeon: The Man Behind the Mask"*, Dr. German gives the reader unique insight into his life and shares with incredible detail personal stories about the journey he took in becoming a doctor and the toll it took on those around him. I felt a range of emotions as I worked my way through his book and gained a powerful new appreciation for the men/women behind the mask. Dr. German is proof that with sheer determination and focus one can accomplish his dreams. He has a unique ability to communicate in a way that the reader will feel that they are right there with him, whether for fishing for lobster in Newfoundland, hitch hiking to a med school interview, exploring a cadaver for the vagus nerve or watching a patient die and knowing there is nothing you can do to change their fate." —John Houseman, educator

"I never knew exactly what it took to be a doctor. Wow!! Now I know! I loved hearing and reading of Dr. German's journey. His humor, insights, and passion for life was incredible to experience. I especially loved reading the intimate details of his surgeries and observations. Congratulations!"
—Cynthia Carney-Potter

"Richard German has written a memoir that exposes the realities of medical education to the outsider. He tells his story with humor and a sharp eye for detail. It is a wonderfully human story, too. The most appealing part is that you get to know Dr. German. There is a fearlessness about the way he works and lives. Maybe that comes with surgery. You get the sense too that this is a good guy. By knowing Dr. German, you come away with a restored faith in the medical profession. If I have to go in for a spleen removal, let it be Dr. German."
—David Holmes, PhD.

"In lively prose, Dr. German's book captures, for the general reader, the essence of the early training of a surgeon—the long hours, tedium, tension and hierarchical structure, as well as the humor, comradeship, exhilaration of correctly applying hard-earned knowledge, and long term satisfaction. More than any other group of physicians, surgeons are faced with situations that require rapid decisions and use of physical skills to prevent disastrous consequences. Dr. German's descriptions of his OR experiences are riveting. A feature of the book that deserves special commendation is the frank descriptions of his life outside of medicine. Dr. German's experiences as an extern in Newfoundland certainly shaped his perspective on medicine and will be of great interest to the public."
–John Edelsberg, M.D.

"I really enjoyed this book! I couldn't put it down! I loved the way it was written, with surgical precision, so that every word counted. Dr. German has given us a wonderful look at the human/emotional side of attending medical school, residency and coming to terms with holding a life in his hands as a surgeon. The book is filled with amusing anecdotes that keep the reader engaged and wanting more." –Bill Potter, businessman

Surgeon:

The Man
Behind the Mask

RICHARD H. GERMAN, M.D., F.A.C.S.

DEDICATION

To Lynn, Lauren and Holly.
Thank you for your love.
I am a blessed man.

SPECIAL THANKS

To my friend Mike Ramsdell who offered me inspiration and encouragement to complete what I started many years ago; to my friend and fellow med student John Edelsberg, M.D. who provided many hours of technical assistance editing and expanding the scope of this book; to Martha Humphreys who was invaluable in helping me dig deeper into my personal emotions and bare my soul; and to Tom Humphreys, a Navy pilot during Viet Nam, who provided accurate military descriptions and technical feedback.

Table of Contents

PREFACE

The moment of truth for any surgeon, the time when he must reach deep down into his soul and draw from his training, experience, imagination, intelligence, and guts, is that precise moment in the operating room when his patient suddenly enters crisis mode, and he stares Death directly in the eye, retina to retina.

For whatever reason, the patient's disease/condition or surgical error, suddenly the surgeon and patient are spiraling down into a black hole. If the patient goes there, he takes his surgeon with him. And the last thing a surgeon wants is to lose control of his patient.

This heart pounding moment, familiar to anyone who has ever held a scalpel over an open body, floods the system with adrenalin that powers the surgeon into focused, top of his game, attention.

Trauma surgeons share this experience more than most.

High risk, Type-A personalities are drawn to this specialty. High risk yields intense reward. However, when ego is trumped by circumstance, one's first instinct is to seek help.

"Houston, we have a problem!"

As a resident, one option was always to stabilize the situation and call for a more experienced advisor.

As a professional, there is no "Houston", only the man behind the mask. Sweating, heart throbbing, eyes wide, brain revved into overdrive, perhaps for a split second distracted by the momentous gravity of the situation, the surgeon calls on every resource he has to transcend personal doubts and insecurities, to intensify his focus and, by God, come up with a solution.

The alternative of witnessing the steady slide toward death is unacceptable. In a perfect world, the surgeon stabilizes the patient and then takes a moment to gather his thoughts before proceeding. Occasionally that pause is so powerful it sometimes means stepping away from the table and leaning against the wall, folding his arms across his chest to take a few deep breaths before returning to his struggle to save the patient.

In a perfect world…

How often does that happen…

Occurring at 1 PM in the afternoon, or more often at 2 AM in the morning, this particular emergency has taken everyone in the room by surprise. The regular "beep-beeps" from the cardiac monitor attest to the patient's viability, a good sign. The stone-cold-silence and frightened stares of the other four people in the room are focused on the surgeon and contributes to the tension. Transcending all of this "noise" is the unbroken creed that the surgeon is responsible, and above all, "First do no harm."

SECTION ONE:

FOUNDATION

CHAPTER ONE

SIDE STEP

*"Nothing of significance has ever been
achieved except by those who knew
that deep inside they were superior
to circumstance."*
Unknown

"Oh! Carol",
Neil Sedaka, 1959

March 19th, 1962

Driving the used car given to us by her parents, I dropped Carol at Vassar to finish her senior year, and then I returned to my junior year at Amherst. The sun was shining, the music on WROC, the Beach Boys' "Little Deuce Coupe" with an incessant rock beat urging me on the road to my future—-no, not only my future, not anymore, now it was **our** future.

My first class of the last semester of my junior year was an American History seminar—the professor and fifteen students. The students sat around an oval table designed to encourage an open exchange of information between us and our professor. Dr. Blakely, PhD was in his early 30's, handsome, trim and totally blind. His first book had just been accepted for publication so he was bubbling with enthusiasm on this spring morning.

"Before we start," he said, "Let's go around the table and hear what each of you did over Spring break. Let's start with you, Tom."

"I went home to Pennsylvania, played some tennis, relaxed."

"Randy?"

"I stayed here on campus, got some studying done, and dropped in on my girlfriend at Holyoke."

"Peter?"

"Spring training with the rugby team and without our best break away..." He tossed me an angry glance.

"Rich?"

"I got married."

Silence.

Dr. Blakely's eyebrows shot up over his sightless eyes, as his mouth formed a perfect "o". He gaped momentarily.

"You got what!?" he stammered. "M-Married?"

"Yes, sir. Carol and I spent our honeymoon on the Cape."

"Well, congratulations!"

"Thank you, sir."

A liberal arts men's college, Amherst was steeped in conservative traditions. Chapel was required three times a week at 7:30 a.m. before classes. Most of the students were WASPs (White Anglo-Saxon Protestants), some Roman Catholics, a pinch of Jews and two blacks in the whole school. Amherst had the infamous "underachiever program" wherein you were required to live up to a certain academic standard (a very specific grade range based on your I.Q., SAT's and relative class standing from high school) or you were expelled. You read it correctly: *EXPELLED!* One student had an 82 GPA and was sent packing for underachieving—administrative expectations were for an 84 to an 89 GPA. These were the dark ages of Amherst academia and are well documented in the archives of Amherst in the '50's and early 60's. As my freshman English professor had told us, "There are only two grades I give out—perfect or fail."

Like a tsunami my unexpected announcement not just on the professor, but on my fellow students as well, washed over the class in a comment smothering wave. On that day, I was the only married student in my class, the youngest married student in college and the only married junior pre-med student the college had ever had.

Today—no big deal.

Back then—a very big deal.

> ## *"Come with me, my love, to the sea, the sea of love...",*
> *"Sea of Love", Phil Phillips, 1959*

Carol and I met when we were sixteen. Lindsey, Carol's roommate at Dana Hall School for Girls near Boston had been my first "girlfriend" growing up. As neighbors, Lindsey and I had fun with childhood games: hide and seek games, climbing trees, roller skating; and I taught her how to shoot my bow and arrow. That had been the extent of my girlfriend experience, not because I wasn't interested in girls, I simply lacked the time or the interest in any one specific girl. That changed the instant I met Carol at our summer cottage on Long Island Sound.

I immediately got lost in her deep, dark brown eyes. Framed by shiny black hair, her perfectly oval face expressed her inquisitive, intelligent mind—a Venus, emerging from the sea, except she was dressed in shorts and a T-shirt, and stood across the lawn from me. Her warm smile indicated she knew a secret that she wanted to share with me, and I couldn't wait to find out what it was...I was hooked on my very first blind date.

> *"When a man loves a woman,*
> *can't keep his mind on nothing else."*
> *"When a Man Loves a Woman",*
> *Percy Sledge, 1966*

As we walked along the beach she shared that secret with me. Giving me words I hadn't heard before—James Joyce, Albert Camus, Feodor Dostoevsky, transcendental existentialism, she expanded my mind with her enthusiasm for the works of these famous writers and thinkers. All of my father's prior efforts to encourage me to read the classics had gone for naught...I wasn't interested. My former life was spent outdoors blue crabbing in the creek using stinky fish heads as bait, building a *Kon Tiki* raft from driftwood logs on the beach and using the faded red and gray awnings discarded from our front porch as a sail. Mowing lawns and washing cars in the summer, shoveling snow in the winter to earn enough money for my first red and white Schwinn bicycle left little time to improve my life through the written word.

Carol's excitement when she discussed their work infected me with a new found interest in ideas and concepts

I had successfully resisted until then. Her face flushed, her expressive hands, communicated the brilliance, the originality, and the unique perspective each great thinker brought to his legacy. I was a blank slate that she apparently enjoyed writing on, as our relationship continued after we returned to our respective prep schools that fall.

We dated through prep school (Suffield Academy in Suffield, Connecticut for me, Dana Hall in Wellesley, Massachusetts for Carol). Dated is a stretch since I saw her only two or three times during the school year, and occasionally on summer weekends when I borrowed Dad's magenta exterior, white interior 1957 Oldsmobile Starfire convertible.

My summer jobs had been day labor in home construction and painting. Paid in cash, which went directly into my pocket on Friday afternoon, then home for a shower and a quick " 'Bye Mom, 'Bye Dad" before I climbed into the car and hit Route 95 to Boston, from our home in Madison, Connecticut to her home in Taunton, Massachusetts 2 ½ hours away. Gas cost 25 cents a gallon, $3 for a tank full, and Mom would always send me off with my "turnpike care package", a tuna and cheese sandwich, chips, Macintosh apple, two homemade chocolate chip cookies and a bottle of Coke. Top down, radio tuned to the "Cousin Brucey" show on 77 AM WABC (NYC), I felt like a big bad dog.

Carol and I would motor out onto Narragansett Bay in her dad's boat, fish and laugh the day away as we fed the swirling, ravenous seagulls that swept off the stern with bits of bait and chips. Saturday evening we packed up the car with goodies, headed for the beach on the Cape with some friends, and steamed little neck clams and lobsters in a boiling pot of fresh seawater over a roaring, snapping fire, made with dried seaweed and ubiquitous driftwood. Our friend played his guitar, and the magical sounds in the dark of night mingled with the ocean waves kicking against the shore and the snapping sea-weed we threw on the fire. I leaned over to Carol and gently licked the warm dribblet of butter on her chin, an inviting residue left over from the last steamed clam she had just eaten. Then off her mouth. Hypnotized by the rising sparks against the dark night sky, and the lingering warm sand against the chill night air, oblivious to everyone else, we rolled up in our blanket and kissed the night away.. We knew life was good.

Once the school year began, our rendezvous were curtailed due to distance and lack of transportation. When the opportunity did arrive, I was fully prepared. Or so I thought. It was Spring Prom at Dana Hall, a must-do event for Carol. I borrowed my Dad's tuxedo and his car for the weekend. What a trusting guy!

Before heading off to Dana Hall, our baseball team had a game at the farthest west end of the state, Kent School at Kent, Connecticut, near the New York state line. I was the first baseman, an average fielder with a Type-A personality and adrenalin to spare; when I connected, the ball disappeared into space. When I missed, the catcher and ump ducked and dove for the dust.

My plan was to drive Dad's car from Suffield to Kent, then from Kent to Dana Hall after the game. Instead, the headmaster, Mr. Appleton Seaverns, who we fondly referred to as "Ap", drove my Dad's car to Kent forcing me to travel with the team on the bus and denying me the fun of a temporary escape in that magenta machine.

Nervously looking at the scoreboard for the time, I watched the score tie at the bottom of the fifth. With only two innings to go, I prayed for a hit—from either team—to avoid any possibility of extra innings. I stared at every batter as they approached the plate. I watched them kick at the dirt in the box, watched them take a few practice swings...then a few more practice swings...then a few more dust kicks...then another glance at the scoreboard for the time...a sigh, and the sad thought I was going to miss the first dance at Carol's prom. Extra innings came and went, until finally, our number 4 batter took a golf swing at Ball Four, and parked it! The home team was three up and three down and I raced into the locker room, took off my cleats, grabbed my duffle bag, and ran in my socks and sweaty uniform to the car which the headmaster had so conveniently (or so I had thought) left for me in front of the gym, keys in the ignition.

Yes! I jumped in and sped off to Dana Hall. I had 200 miles on the Mass Turnpike to contort myself and change out of my uniform and into my tux, all the while driving the car with my knee caps on the steering wheel. I can only imagine what the passing cars must have thought I was doing, elbows flying and weaving back and forth in my lane. A spritz of Old Spice after shave every 50 miles assured a warm reception.

Carol's smile of relief at my appearance chased the stress away. The dance had already started, and the circle of couples was surrounded by a ring of Puritanical school-marms with mouse grey hair in tight curls or a tighter bun at the base of their necks and piercing stares behind their prim and proper glasses. The only privacy was found in the center of the circle, duck down and make out like crazy until another amorous couple bumped us back to the outside of the circle. Once the dance was over, the girls were dutifully escorted back to their dorm rooms. Period. End of report.

When I arrived at Suffield Sunday evening, my roommate rushed up to the car and said, "Rich, get to Ap's office, pronto!"

"What's wrong?" I asked.

"You were supposed to drive Ap back here from Kent after the game! You split so fast he ended up on the team bus!"

"I'm screwed."

Terrified for my future at Suffield, I cautiously tapped on his office door.

"Come in, Richard."

My heart pounded. My palms sweat. My knees knocked, as that earlier pot I was watching on the beach boiled over with the realization that suddenly I was dead meat—a cooked, bright red lobster—a goner, expelled!

Ap was puffing on his pipe, pushed back from his desk in a relaxed posture, his demeanor was pleasant, not that of an executioner.

"Richard, I can forgive you for leaving me stranded in Kent, but I cannot forgive you going to the Dana Hall Spring Prom without a shower!"

He nodded his head and smiled.

"And I expect an excellent grade on your Algebra exam tomorrow."

"Yes, sir. Thank you, sir."

What a guy! What a man! When I entered Suffield, Ap had commented that he had great expectations for me.

I was not about to let him down. And I earned an excellent grade, indeed.

The fall of my senior year in prep school finally arrived. Carol was a freshman at Vassar though we saw very little of each other during the school year. It was time to apply for college and I had my top three choices all lined up. By tradition, Ap personally interviewed each senior (only 52 of us in my entire class) to "aid" in the students' aspirations, i.e. if you were a "C" student, you didn't apply to Harvard. I stood outside Ap's office patiently waiting for an invitation into the inner-sanctum. The door opened, a fellow senior exited with a smile on his face, and I was up next.

"Come in, Richard," Ap directed.

He was seated at his polished mahogany desk, neat as a pin, with my academic records in front of him. Smoke curled up from his well-worn pipe.

"Sit down, Richard and tell me what your choices are for college."

"Well, sir, I have applications to Williams, Dartmouth and Cornell," I said confidently.

"Those are all fine choices," Ap replied. "You will do very well at Amherst. You are especially good in math. It's a better school for you."

"But, sir, what do I do with these applications?" I asked.

"Just leave them with me, Richard. You'll be receiving your acceptance to Amherst shortly," Ap said with complete composure. And just like that, my future had been determined by one man. One hell of a man. I would not disappoint him.

"In My Room",
The Beach Boys, 1963

My first two years at Amherst were challenging. Physics, math, English, French, humanities and history— all freshman required courses, four credits each. A real ball buster with sports crammed into each season. Advanced physics, calculus, bio-chem and inorganic and analytic chemistry filled my sophomore year when I beat out the senior wrestler for the 177 pound slot on the wrestling team. I felt badly for the guy—he was captain, but ended up sitting on the bench while I wrestled in his place. But not so badly that I was going to give into anyone.

Carol and I saw each other on scattered occasions, mostly during the summer when I would drive up for a weekend in my dad's car from our summer home in Madison to Taunton, just south of Boston. But then there was that rare opportunity during the school year when sports worked to my advantage. I was a junior; she was a senior. On the wrestling team since my junior year in prep school, I was now the team captain at Amherst. The distance factor and the academic demands of a pre-med at Amherst playing three sports a year helped to put a damper on our relationship. Having no mode of transportation other than a bicycle did not help any. The opportunity came when our wrestling team went to Williams College for a meet in early December. Williamstown is a small college town nestled in far western Massachusetts near the New York border and 85 miles closer to Vassar. Williams' mascot was a purple cow (believe it or not!) and Amherst's mascot was Lord Jeffrey Amherst, a soldier of King George II of England, and for whom our college was named in 1821.

That day Lord Jeff "milked" the purple cow and I won my match by a pin in the second 3 minute period. After we took victorious showers, the team left by bus back to Amherst and I left by thumb down to Vassar in a late afternoon New England blizzard. Three Williams college students picked me up. They were stinking of beer, had just left a fraternity party and were attempting to navigate the slippery mountain roads of Williamstown. We quickly spun off the road and into a snow bank. I got out of the car and offered to help shovel them out. Waving me off, the three "purple cows" cracked open another beer from their well-stocked cooler and began to sing college songs, happy to be stuck in the snow. So I put on a smile and stuck out my thumb again. The next ride carried me all the way to Albany in three hours, then down to Poughkeepsie in a truck.

Christmas was a welcome break from the Amherst pre-med grind—a little skiing, a little sleep, a little Carol. Her birthday was on Christmas Day so we schlepped down to New York City and stayed with my sister Anne and her fiancé Bill on the East Side. NYC was not my cup of tea— too crowded, too rushed, too pushy. Give me a romp in the Connecticut woods and, as Robert Frost wrote, let me be a swinger of birches. In fact, I always felt a bit insecure in that enclosure of concrete, glass and steel. I certainly appreciate how grating, loud, hectic and yes, exciting for some, a big city can be. I appreciate that aspect of life, that high level of energy and interaction that feeds the soul of many. On the other hand, I found my soul in the solitude of nature, and since I was a young boy I always sought comfort in the shadow of maples and oaks, or digging for little neck clams in Madison on the rocky shoals revealed at low tide. That was my escape—my security.

Too soon, too soon, Christmas break was over and there I was in bio-chem lab dreaming of what road less travelled by that I would eventually take in life. But I was disturbed—somehow, some way I was losing that special feeling for Carol, that intensity that used to keep me thinking of her all the time. Now I was checking out some of the Smith and Mt. Holyoke girls who wandered through my fraternity house in T-shirts and jeans, or T-shirts and no jeans. Carol had been my one and only girlfriend, but temptation was creeping into my jeans and I could not help but envy my Theta Delta Chi fraternity brothers who would parade a seemingly endless troop of college betties up and down the stairs for enhancement of their carnal knowledge. One of my roommates (five of us in one room, double bunks, so as to spare the other two rooms for "entertainment") named Mike kept goading me to start dating.

"Rich, my girlfriend is bringing her roommate Vickie to the house party this weekend. I think you two should connect."

"I don't know, Mike. I'll have to see how I feel. No commitment", I responded.

"Rich, Carol is 150 miles away at Vassar. You never see her 'cause you play sports every damn weekend and you have no transportation. Getting laid now and then is not all that bad! You're spending too much time reading Playboy!"

"Gee, thanks for the advice, Mike. Remember, no commitment".

"O.K., O.K.", he replied.

Saturday Amherst hosted MIT in wrestling. I faced a tough opponent, and in keeping with my usual pre-match habit, I holed up alone in a friend's room for thirty minutes, sitting on his bed, nearly hypnotized listening to

Buddy Holly's song "Rave On" over and over and over. It was a ritual that everyone respected, and no one ever disturbed me while I got into my warm-up trance. By the time I walked on to the wrestling mat, I was in a different zone, impervious to outside influences, riveted on my opponent and unbeatable (all but twice). Amherst lost, but I won my match. I became known as something just short of maniacal, but I could hear the fans stomping their feet in unison on the wooden bleachers and it sent my adrenaline into overdrive. What a rush! To this day, no sport has so excited me as wrestling, mano-a-mano. You victor or you don't and it's all up to you. Of course, that was the essence of my very Dutch upbringing. "Win or lose, Butch," my dad would say, "it's up to you."

The match was over by 4 p.m. I showered, crammed down a burger and went back to Theta Delt and crashed.

"German, German, I've been looking for you!"

Mike was shaking my bed like a 6.8 earthquake.

"It's 9 o'clock. The party's raging downstairs! Beer and betties galore! And Susan's friend is dying to meet you."

"I don't know, Mike. I'm beat. I had a tough match today."

"German, if you don't come down and meet this girl I'm bringing her up here! Now get your ass in gear."

"All right, all right, Mike. Give me five."

I threw on a sweatshirt, jeans and loafers and made my way down into the den of inequity, bumper to bumper frat brothers and babes, the stale smell of spilled beer on the wood floor that stuck to your shoes and juke box banging out vibes. It was like a mating ritual. All of these highly intelligent students, proven exceptional exam takers—all in the hunt for very basic reasons.

"German, over here", Mike was screaming.

I made my way through a pack of over-heated bodies all gyrating in unison.

"Hi, Mike", I said.

"German, I want you to meet Vickie."

"Hi, Vickie."

Mike was right—she was slender, stacked, long dark hair, blue eyes.

"Do I call you 'German'?" she asked.

"No. Rich is better."

"Well, Rich, what do you say we dance?"

She grabbed me just as my favorite song came on the jukebox—Ray Charles' "Georgia on My Mind".

In place of bodies crashing like atoms in a Bohr Chamber, everyone morphed into the next part of the mating ritual—moaning and grinding. My heart was pounding as Vickie was communicating her intentions in very creative ways. She looked up at me and we kissed. Everyone was kissing, or grinding, or something. And I was getting a chubby to boot.

"Rich, take me upstairs."

On my God! What do I do? A swirl of conflicting emotions was flooding my brain, but my hormones were definitely leading me in one direction. Steam was starting to rise. Then out of the blue, I thought I heard something.

"German, German!"

Over the din of music, moans and groans, I barely heard my name being called from someone upstairs. But this time it was louder and more emphatic.

"GERMAN! You've got a phone call!"

"What the shit! What's this all about?" I thought to myself.

"Vickie, I'll be right back."

"Rich, hurry!"

I ran up the stairs, two at a time. The only phone in the fraternity house, a pay phone, was in a small cubicle next to the mail room. I grabbed the phone which had been left hanging by the cord.

"Hello?" I asked.

"Rich, I had to call you."

It was Carol. Her voice was quivering.

"I'm pregnant."

"Oh, my God! Are you sure?" I asked in disbelief.

"I saw the doctor today. I'm pregnant."

Silence. I was dumbfounded. My heart was pounding—this time from shock and the unknown.

"What do we do?" I asked, searching for an answer, looking for guidance.

"I don't know, Rich. Let's both think about it. Call me tomorrow."

I felt like throwing up. I put on my heavy Amherst jacket, walked out into the winter snow and didn't come back for two hours.

The next day Mike gave me shit for leaving Vickie in heat but that was the last thing on my mind. I had a physics exam coming up, a pregnant girlfriend at Vassar and no car to get down there. The following Saturday was free, and I hooked a ride with a nerdy classmate who was dating a plain-Jane girl at Vassar. Not my idea of a fun trip to Poughkeepsie, but it beat the hell out of hitch-hiking for four hours. I pretended I was tired, and closed my eyes for most of the drive, as much to avoid stupid conversation as to think about what I was going to say to Carol.

I met Carol in the main lobby of her dorm, took her hand and sat down in the most secluded part of the adjacent study. Her dark, beautiful eyes were looking at me in anticipation.

"Carol, I think we should get married," I almost whispered.

"Rich, I was hoping you would say that."

What a way to propose to a woman. I was scared to death, not at all sure of what we were doing, no ring to offer, and definitely not down on one knee. We kissed gently and that was that. No tears of joy, no great relief. More a sense of resignation and acceptance.

The next weekend Carol came up to watch me wrestle at Wesleyan University in my hometown of Middletown, Connecticut. This, of course, was planned and Mom and Dad came to watch as well. I lost my match to Jim Ferguson, a black star athlete on scholarship who went to the NCAA Nationals and came in ninth in the nation. Still, I was disappointed. After the match, Mom and Dad tried to comfort me for my loss, but by my subdued behavior they sensed something else was wrong. When we got home, Carol went into the living room as planned.

"Mom, Dad, can I talk with you?"

They froze. The three of us went into their bedroom and they immediately sat down on the edge of the bed in stiff anticipation. The air was so thick you could cut it with your hand. My heart was racing, my face flushed, by ears burning, my gut churning.

"Carol and I are getting married", I announced in a tone that lacked joy or conviction. Dad immediately responded, "Are you already married?" (meaning pregnant).

"Yes, Dad, we are."

Mom started crying and Dad got tears in his eyes, an uncommon display of emotion for him. Mom sobbed, "But Richard, what about your dream to become a doctor? Is that over now?"

"No, Mom, I will become a doctor."

Dad interrupted, "How could you do this to me?" As an immigrant from Holland, Dad was always insecure about his image in American society.

I swallowed hard. "Dad, I'm sorry."

"Well, Richard, your mother and I will support you," my dad responded in his usual stoic manner.

By that time Carol had come into the bedroom and we were all crying. We hugged, dried our tears and right then and there all four of our lives changed forever.

As for my sister Anne, that was a whole different story. Expecting understanding and support from one's own sister was not unreasonable, especially since we had been close as kids. She was protective of me, her younger brother, until I didn't need protection anymore, evidently.

"Well, Richard, you've made your bed, now you get to sleep in it!" was her comment to me. I was stunned and embarrassed. I felt gut punched again. Blind sided. Out of the blue, her demeanor had totally changed. No sympathy in her voice, no warmth, no compassion. "Where in the hell did that come from?" I wondered, and I lived with it in silence until Mom offered an explanation years later. Sibling rivalry had reared its ugly head. Anne, the older child, was meant to marry first, get pregnant first and produce the first grandchild. And I had gotten in the way.

Carol and I had planned our wedding to take place in her hometown of Taunton, Massachusetts over Spring break. Carol told her parents of her pregnancy. Her mom was

O.K.—her dad not so O.K. He and I never hit it off very well but to his credit he supported us and gave us a car to use.

The wedding was on a beautiful, warmish Saturday in mid-March 1962. A thin crowd of six showed up—both sets of parents, Carol and I. Dad and I had a moment alone on the steps outside the First Parish Unitarian Church before the ceremony. In rare form, Dad reached out to me in a personal way and asked, "Rich, are you sure you're O.K. with this?" Jesus Christ! What a time and place for my dad to ask me such a question. Yet another gut punch. I never thought I had any option to this marriage thing, and now Dad was testing my resolve on the church steps?

"Sure, Dad, I'm O.K.".

Twenty minutes later, Carol and I walked down those same steps as Mr. and Mrs. Richard German.

"There's a summer place...."
Theme from "A Summer Place",
Percy Faith Orchestra, 1960

The honeymoon cottage, a loaner from Charlie and Ginny Collins, close friends of Carol's parents, was among a sprinkling of summer homes, nestled near the sand dunes and waving sea grass, so typical in the Cape. Populated to distraction in the summer, but nearly deserted in March, the Cape was delightfully quiet.

In addition to the crisp, new $100 bill from the Collins, a fortune to me, we were thrilled to discover the fridge already stocked with little neck clams, two cooked, bright red 1 ¾ pound lobsters, a bottle of cold sparkling Burgundy, butter, eggs and everything else we would need for an amorous, romantic weekend.

Our first morning as a married couple, Carol and I woke to the sounds of seagulls. Carol had fixed us a fabulous breakfast of crisp, thick bacon, scrambled eggs mixed with peppers and onions, warm scones with fresh, Cape Cod blackberry jam and hot, steaming coffee. If this was married life, then I was one very lucky man. I grabbed the morning paper, a second cup of coffee and went outside and sat on the porch steps to enjoy the warming sun.

Having been brought up in Oak Bluffs on Martha's Vineyard (discovered by the English explorer Bartholomew Gosnold in 1602 and named in honor of his mother-in-law or his daughter who died in infancy, both named Martha), my dear mother always described such a day as a "Vineyard Day". This was a generic term for a beautiful, crisp, bright blue sunny day that would bless us in late spring or early fall. Such a day made you feel so very privileged to be alive and witness the sparkles dancing wildly off the blue ocean, gray-wing-tipped, bone white seagulls banking slowly in the air to survey the aquatic menu beneath them.

Engrossed in an article about President Kennedy, I slowly became aware of the soft crunching sound of wheels across gravel drawing closer. I looked up to an unusual sight—an octogenarian sitting in a wheel chair and his caretaker beside him, about thirty feet down the walkway. His nurse was tall, perhaps 5' 10", stoutly built and wore a starched white mid-calf length uniform with endless buttons up the front, white hose and white, thick-heeled shoes. Her dark brown hair was drawn up in a tight bun and she performed her duty in precise, terse New England tradition. Her job, this bright, beautiful, warm Cape Cod day, was to wheel her charge out for "morning air".

Carol came out to join me on the steps and we must have appeared just as unusual to them. He waved and directed his nurse to wheel him closer.

"Good morning, sir." I said respectfully.

"Well, a good morning to you, too", he responded, his deep voice phlegmy with age. "And who might you be? Are you friends of Charlie and Ginny?"

"As a matter of fact, we are. I'm Richard and this is my wife, Carol, from Taunton. We're on our honeymoon, on our spring break from college."

His mouth dropped open. We were both 21 years-old but looked more like 18 or 19.

"But you're just kids. You must be younger than my grandchildren!" He coughed to catch his breath. "What are your plans after college?"

Apparently he couldn't get over it, his deeply veined hands plucked at the Campbell tartan blanket covering his knees. He shook his head in disbelief or perhaps it was just a touch of palsy that comes with age.

"I plan to become a doctor, a surgeon." My voice reflected a confidence I did not feel when speaking to this elderly gentleman. At that time I was still over six months away from even applying to medical school...without any guarantees that I would be accepted.

He squinted slightly, adjusted the plaid blanket lying across his lap and looked back at me, his rheumy blue eyes wide with poorly restrained disbelief.

"Richard, you'll never make it . . . ."

His tone did not reflect an opinion, but rather a prediction, more representative of his generational thinking than an insult to mine.

CHAPTER TWO

PRE-MED, MARRIAGE and MY MISSION

"We must believe that we are gifted for something, and that this thing, whatever the cost, must be attained."
Marie Curie, physicist and chemist

"That'll be the Day,"
Buddy Holly, 1958

Suppressing the elderly man's concerns from my brand new bride, I walked into the kitchen, turned on A.M. Radio Boston and "That'll Be the Day..." played from the small portable on the counter.

"That I'll say good-bye..." to my plans of med school and a career in medicine. I thought of the irony of my recent conversation and then the vote of confidence from Buddy Holly.

Carol's voice interrupted by musings. "What's the matter, Rich?"

"Nothing, honey." I took her hand and we walked outside. "Don't worry. We'll make it."

"What? Me worry?" she said, quoting a popular saying of Alfred E. Newman of Mad Magazine. "Not a chance!" She smiled and we embraced. We both needed each other's tacit assurance. The strength of her arms around me indicated she was telling me the truth.

We made a small picnic lunch of leftover cold, steamed clams, fresh bread, fruit and cheese and two bottles of Coke. Genius that I was, I figured it would be fun to take the dirt road down to the beach. The not-so-genius part was driving the car off the dirt road into the sand, effectively immobilizing us, all four wheels worth.

Try finding a shovel, two long 2 x 6 wood planks and some plywood on a deserted road off of a deserted beach in a near deserted village during off-season Cape Cod. I scavenged the necessary equipment, assembled them at the car and started digging.

Carol, God bless her, was supportive and pitched in to help. I was embarrassed, then angry, then determined. There was no AAA, no gas station, no tow truck. There was Rich German and two hours of digging which finally resulted in backing the car onto the dirt road—terra firma!

Sandy, sweaty and stinky, we sat on a blanket near a sand dune and the razor sharp, light green dune grass, a soft breeze blowing the seagulls around, and ate clams to our hearts' delight. Step by step, I thought. That's how I dug myself out of the sand, that's how I'm going to reach my goal.

Carol and I threw the Frisbee around and ran in the soft, fine sand of Cape Cod. The water was too cold for swimming so we sat in our shorts and sweaters on the beach and dug our feet into the warmish sand. Moments like these caused an occasional twinge of guilt that I had taken time out from academia and college routine, that I was playing while the rest of the world was slowly spinning and progressing, leaving me behind.

As long as I could remember, even as a kid, I felt uncomfortable if I wasn't being productive. New England puritanical work ethic combined with my Dutch heritage carried me forward into adulthood. As a second grader, when my best friend, David Eaton, received a brand new red and white Schwinn bicycle for his 7th birthday, I wanted one, too. It had shiny chrome handlebars, a headlight on the front fender, black handgrips with red and white plastic streamers, a loud ringing bell, red reflectors on the back fender, and most important, the letters *SCHWINN* emblazed along the middle bar. Breathless with envy, I went running to my dad to make my request. Dad gazed at me with that stern, Dutch look, curled his right index finger, beckoning me to follow him into the garage. He pointed to the lawn mower and said, "There's your Schwinn bicycle, Butch".

Thus began my first earning experience. I had the use of the lawn mower for free, room and board included, no advertising expenses, no worker's compensation insurance costs, and when I stubbed my toe on a rock, my mom applied ice and a band-aid so I needed no health insurance. All payment was in cash and I paid no taxes. 100% profit. What a great business model! Even a seven year-old could succeed!

My father was born in Amsterdam, Netherlands in 1909, the second oldest of seven brothers and sisters. After World War I devastated Europe, my grandparents Oma and Opa collected their brood and sailed for Ellis Island.

Opa found work as a mechanic in a very poor neighborhood in East Hartford, Connecticut. At first he worked on automobiles and later on complex machinery at the Sikorsky Helicopter installation in Hartford. His mechanical genius was instrumental in the war effort during World War II. A martinet, Opa was a physically strict disciplinarian and penurious to a fault. The soul of the family, Oma nurtured the children and taught them life's great lessons. Imbuing a sense of achievement in my father, her positive influence flowed down upon me.

One day, when I was seven or eight years old, my father took me aside, a rare event in itself, and spoke to me from the "gospel according to Oma": "Richard, I was given a platform by Oma and Opa on which to start my life. It is my responsibility to elevate myself from this platform to a higher level. You have the privilege of starting at a higher level than I did, and the responsibility of raising yourself even higher, and, in turn, pass this tradition on to your children when the time comes."

Although, he never repeated these words to me, they have remained deeply embedded in my psyche ever since. When the ocean of my life picks up with fair winds and following seas, or boils with riptides and 12 foot waves, those words have always shone like a beacon from a lighthouse (located) at True North.

So how could I possibly feel guilty on my honeymoon? I guess the old man's words left me a little insecure, and

being the only married pre-med student at Amherst added
to the challenge.

I played three sports each year throughout college—
football, wrestling and rugby. At 6 feet 1 inches, 185
pounds, I was always in good shape. I never smoked and
only drank an occasional back-East gin and tonic during off
season or summer time. Wrestling was an intense discipline, a very individual sport that gave one great personal
satisfaction and victory, even if the team lost—no question
this was a sport of you first, and the team second. If you
did well, the team benefited. Amherst was not known as a
wrestling powerhouse but the sport taught me some great
principles that have stayed with me.

On the other hand, rugby was a "balls-to-the-wall"
springtime sport, a free-for-all, organized chaos with a
wonderful opportunity to ad-lib tackles, play two 30
minute non-stop periods and leave all your aggressions on
the field. And believe it or not, tiny Amherst (total of
1,200 men and no women), in 1963, *was* a rugby powerhouse. We beat N.Y. Rugby Club, Dartmouth, Brown,
Wesleyan and Williams. Our only defeat was to Harvard
6 to 3. The team was in spring training in Ft. Lauderdale,
Florida, while I was on my honeymoon.

"Thank Heaven for Little Girls",
Maurice Chevalier, 1958

After a week on the Cape, it was time to get back to
reality. I returned to Amherst after dropping Carol off at
Vassar to finish up her senior year as a drama major. Carol
felt that the honest and right thing to do would be to
request a change in her student status to "married". She

was confronted by Vassar President Sarah Gibson Blanding (SGB) as to the circumstances of this change in status. The explosive result was that Carol was summarily ejected from Vassar two months prior to graduation. In spite of honor grades as a superlative student, this repudiation was outrageous, but our society was on the very cusp of transition from a disposition steeped in a Puritanical-Victorian mentality to the liberal tsunami that gained momentum by the late 1960's to the norm we accept today. Obviously, Vassar rejected the concept of pre-marital sex. God forbid that a pregnant-appearing graduate in cap and gown would cast an aspersion on the pristine reputation of a "Vassar girl".

I wrote a letter of protest to SGB, predictably to no avail. In retrospect, SGB missed a classic opportunity to emerge as a vanguard in women's liberation and become a hero to all women, pregnant or not. Instead, the honorable but petrified SGB withdrew to the safe-zone of her entrenched mentality and fumed in the mundane morass of her starchy tradition. Tough to break inertia and be a leader.*

*On April 4, 1962, in an all campus meeting, SGB told the 1,450 students of Vassar College that pre-marital sex, and excessive drinking would not be tolerated by the college. She explained that disciplinary action would be taken against those who did not follow the standard of the college, for she believed that sexual promiscuity was "indecent and immoral". President Blanding advised those students who could not follow the rules to withdraw voluntarily from Vassar. (Vassar History 1962-1963; faculty.vassar. edu./daniels1962_1963). To Vassar's credit, Carol completed her courses and received her degree from Vassar in May, 2005.

We moved into the Middletown house during the summer months while Mom and Dad went to the Madison cottage as usual. We were only 25 miles apart, but for the first summer of my life I was not living at the shore and the memories of the beach, Long Island Sound and the sea tugged at my heart strings. Regrets? Not really, only the bittersweet nostalgia for what once was...so I turned the car radio to the Beach Boys and imagined those California beaches on my way to one of my various summer jobs.

Since I was ten years old, my summer jobs were usually out of doors and varied: mowing lawns, first by hand mower and then graduating to a power mower, as long as I paid for the gas; painting the neighbors' boardwalks across the marsh down to the sand in varying shades of gray only, as dictated by the rigid rules of the beach members' association; collecting garbage at Hammonasset State Park; picking corn, strawberries and snap peas at Mr. Johnson's farm on the other side of the New York-New Haven railroad tracks that carried folks into the "Big City"; pumping gas at Aidee Bassett's gas station on Main Street and washing down the endless yellow school buses starting on the bus roof on hot summer days where I felt like a bug in a frying pan; waiting on tables on Fisher's Island at an old New England home converted into a funky restaurant and bar downstairs and a hot, sweaty bedroom cot in the attic where I slept, all while the 40-ish husband and wife owners were having separate affairs with the wealthy clientele from Delaware; hanging tobacco high up in the eaves of 40 foot-tall tobacco sheds in northern Connecticut—I was the "hangman" since I had no fear of heights and would balance on beams while hanging yardsticks of sticky tobacco leaves overhead—the tobacco juice trickled down my arms and back, leaving tracks of sweat and barn dust in their wake; painting houses and doing general grunt construction work for Millard's Contractor in Madison.

Now that I was a married man with a baby on the way, I had to make some real dough. I joined the Pipe Cover's Union and insulated the aluminum air conditioning ducts high up on scaffolding for the new gymnasium being built at Wesleyan University in Middletown. The money was grand, and we spent weekends with Mom and Dad, sitting on the beach and walking the sandbars during the day, enjoying cocktail hour in the evening on the gray wood-planked porch overlooking Long Island Sound.

As good as it sounds, I had deep-seated doubts about our future, all three of us. What if I didn't get into med school, and how could I pay for it if I did?

Suddenly it was September, and time to get back to Amherst. Mom and Dad moved back to the Middletown house and Carol and I drove to her parents' house in Taunton where she would stay until the baby was born. I lingered to the last possible moment, and then drove to Amherst.

The moment I arrived on campus four hours later, I called Carol. Her brother told me she was in labor at Boston Lying-In Hospital. So, I turned around and drove back to Boston where I arrived at 1:00 a.m. Our beautiful daughter Lynn arrived at 4 a.m. In those days, fathers were not welcome in the delivery room. So like the others in the waiting room, I paced back and forth until the nurse came out holding Lynn wrapped in a pink blanket. I was overwhelmed. Wow! I'm a dad! Carol had endured 10 hours of tough labor, but was in good spirits, and we were blessed with a healthy baby girl.

As any parent will tell you, your life changes radically the moment your first child is born. After the first warm wave of love at the sight of your child, comes the cold water of responsibility and the realization this small, defenseless child is totally dependent upon you for food, shelter, and survival. The experience took my breath away... momentarily. I watched Carol with our daughter, and when my wife looked at me with those trusting brown eyes, I inhaled her confidence in me and that our future was secure.

"Fun, Fun, Fun",
The Beach Boys, 1964

I drove back to Amherst the next day, prepared the small, 4th floor apartment we had rented above the House of Walsh men's clothier in Amherst Village, and drove back to pick up Carol and Lynn two weeks later.

Our life at Amherst began on the run.

For the first time in my life, I was paying for rent, utilities, groceries and diapers. God Bless my dad, who paid my tuition, and Carol's dad who donated the car. After playing for 6 years, I quit football and took over the food concession selling hot dogs and cokes at the football games. Carol sat in the bleachers cheering the Lord Jeffs. Two month old Lynn slept in the back seat of our car which I had parked next to the concession stand so that I could keep an eye on her while working. Nestled among hot dog buns and mustard containers, angel that she was, Lynn never made a peep during the game.

It was strange selling hot dogs instead of playing in the game catching footballs and making touchdowns for the team I had captained. But the hot dog sales from one game paid for one months' rent ($50) and food ($7 a week) and extras—not bad.

And so started my senior year.

CHAPTER THREE

THE INTERVIEW: THE CRUCIBLE

"Opportunities are seldom labeled"
John Shedd, *author*

"Be True to Your School",
The Beach Boys, 1963

It was October of my senior year at Amherst, and time to consider my options for medical school. The application process preceded the interview… if the application made it that far. I selected the recipients with great care paying attention to the quality of the institution, percentages of wannabe doctors they graduated, and lastly, where those doctors went for their internship. I narrowed my selections to the University of Rochester (my hope) and the University of Albany (my ace in the hole) and sent off my applications together with a check for $35.00 each (one month's groceries) to the admissions offices. Two applications were all I could afford, so I chose carefully.

Once the applications were submitted, there was nothing else to do other than race to the mailbox and look for an appropriate envelope asking for an interview. Work, studies, work, family, work, studies, family took up every spare second, so there was no time to worry about the "if", so I focused on the "when".

Several weeks later, driving through downtown Amherst, I heard an ominous rattle, then a louder "thud", and finally a hiss and my trusty rusty steed came to a completely silent stop in the middle of a left turn at the busiest intersection in this college town. After pushing it to the side of the road, I started to look around for a repair garage, gas station, or tow truck to haul my very fragile Ford in for repairs…again. Why didn't I pay closer attention when Opa showed me how an engine worked? Perhaps I should have skipped college all together and gone to a good mechanic's school. How different could it be replacing engine parts than fixing people's parts? I hoped I lived long enough to find out.

Probably at the exact moment my car died, the admissions counselor licked the stamp on the letter requesting an interview with me in Rochester, 325 miles away.

The car was still in the shop for repairs when the day arrived for my interview, so I hitchhiked from Massachusetts to Rochester, New York. I got a ride to the Mass Turnpike, stuck my thumb out and hoped for someone going my way. I tried not to think about the time, and how long it would take to hitchhike to the interview.

If weather was any indication, the odds were in my favor. The bright pale yellow sunshine of a typical mid-November day in New England highlighted the reds, oranges, deep yellow of the maple, oak and sycamore leaves still on the trees or in piles on the lawns on my route. Crisp oxygen, cindery smell of burning leaves and early fires in fireplaces in the nearby neighborhood invigorated me as I made my way to my favorite pick up point.

Luck was with me, since a sedan stopped for me almost as soon as I turned to stick out my thumb. The salesman was going as far as Albany and wanted some company to keep him awake. His monologue about wife, family, football, almost lulled me to sleep, since my input to the conversation was restricted to an occasional "Oh?" "Really?" "Sure…"

The second ride in a station wagon driven by a middle aged woman took me all the way into Rochester. Her questions as she drove renewed any nerves I thought I had left behind in Massachusetts. After learning of my mission, admission to medical school, she turned and smiled in disbelief.

"You're not wearing those clothes to an interview, are you?" Her eyebrow shot up beneath the wing-tipped frames of her glasses.

"Uh, no ma'am," I responded, raising my travel bag. "My good clothes are in here."

"That's good," she said, returning her attention to the highway. "You don't get second chances to make a good first impression."

Great, I thought, another vote of confidence by a total stranger. She drove out of her way to drop me at a gas station two blocks from the university hospital. "Good luck on your interview!" she said, as she pulled away.

My pre-interview nerves burst forth with renewed energy as I asked the high school dropout female attendant for the key to the men's room. Without looking up, cracking her gum as she read the latest issue of Photoplay, the teenager reached behind her, grabbed the stick with the key on it and held it out toward me.

"Thanks," I said, heading out the door and around the corner to the men's room.

Breathing through my mouth in a futile attempt to not smell the bathroom's filthy interior, I almost tripped over a faded blue mechanic's jacket lying on the grease-stained floor, just inside the door. I picked it up and hung it on a hook. The pungent odor of the camphor block stuck to the white porcelain of the urinal did not quite hide the smell of urine, old cigarette smoke, and something particularly rotten a recent patron had left in the barrel trash can in the corner. And of course, the heat was turned up to steaming.

Working quickly, I took off my shoes, stood in my socks and pulled off my jeans. Not wanting to drag my new khaki pants through the grease on the tile floor, I stood up on the toilet seat in my underwear. Balancing precariously, I carefully pulled my pants on, standing first on one leg, then on the other and jumped down. Almost done...

Feeling flop sweat trickling down my sides, I proudly pulled out a clean white shirt from my duffle bag, buttoned it up, turned and looked in the mirror.

"Jesus Christ!!"

My red face over my bright white shirt...with two large black grease finger prints around the buttons...stared in horror back at me. For a split second I considered trying to scrub them off with the sliver of hand soap swimming in the metal ashtray next to the grimy sink. Since the soap had horizontal lines of black dirt ground into what was left of the bar, I dismissed this idea instantly.

Grumbling, mumbling invectives and really pissed off at myself for picking up that damned mechanic's jacket, I washed my hands once, twice and three times before putting on my tie. Adjusting it to strategically cover the random grease marks with maximum effect, I stretched tall, slumped over, twisted and turned to see if my carelessness was visible. Shrugging in resignation, I yanked at a rough paper towel from the dispenser and covered the door handle with it before opening it to proceed to my interview.

"Walk Like a Man",
Four Seasons, 1963

Bright sunshine warmed my back as I walked briskly to the University Hospital and my interview.

The nine story yellow brick building filled an entire city block. Young men in scrubs, women in a variety of nurses' caps from their nursing schools, delivery men with flowers for a patient, visitors, guests, and out-patients scurried back and forth through the swinging glass doors into the lobby. I held the door for a middle aged woman dragging a child into the main entrance.

As soon as I inhaled that hospital smell I was no longer grumbling and pissed off—I was nervous as hell.

This was the big leagues and my future, I hoped.

I entered the admissions office just as the secretary glanced at the round institutional clock on the off-white walls of the waiting room.

"Mr. German?" she asked, with a smile.

"Yes, ma'am!" I felt like I was reporting for duty.

Her slight resemblance to my favorite aunt relaxed me immediately.

"You're right on time," she commented, handing me a folder to carry into the interviews.

"Thank God since I hitchhiked here."

Her mouth fell open in apparent surprise. What?! Thumbed a ride all the way from Amherst for this interview?"

I nodded and watched the smile return to her face as she rose to pat me on my back as I went through the door behind her into the inner sanctum of the admission officers...all three of them.

The three interviews were over almost before I realized it. Intimidating but manageable, I exited their offices and waited until I entered the waiting room to exhale.

"How'd it go?" the admissions secretary asked.

"Good...I think," I said smiling in relief, if not in confidence in my performance.

"If you have the energy and commitment to hitchhike all that way and face those three curmudgeons," she said, "then you have the stamina to make it through med school."

"Thank you!"

"Oh, and I like your tie."

That made my day!

"It's My Party",
Leslie Gore, 1963

Two months later, mid-January, was big day for us.

It was late afternoon and darkness arrived early. I returned home from wrestling practice and looked forward to a warm bath and warm dinner.

"Hi, honey, how's the baby?"

"She's asleep," Carol replied. "Isn't she precious?"

A rhetorical question.

Looking down at our daughter in her crib, I silently renewed my commitment to our future. I leaned over and kissed Lynn's forehead, dewy with sleep.

"Honey, I'm going to take a long, hot bath." I said, straightening up.

"Okay, take your time. I'll get supper ready."

We had no shower, just a vintage white cast iron, claw foot bathtub. That night the warm water felt especially good as it rose around me in the tub. I put a wash cloth over my face and steeped in the luxury of embryonic-like immersion.

The phone rang.

I heard Carol say, "Western Union?"

An edge of fear tinged her next question. "Can you read it to me? I'm his wife."

Carol squealed and raced into the bathroom.

"Rich! You've been accepted to Rochester!"

Thank God, thank God! Carol leaned over and reached into the bathwater, sleeves and all, to give me a big hug and kiss. She was soaked but who cared! I slipped under the water, holding my breath for a time, in a futile attempt at restraining my emotion. *We're safe, we're going to make it. Thank you, dear Lord,* I thought.

The only obstacle was hard work.

I was meant for hard work.

Fall turned into winter and I looked forward to wrestling season. The training, the discipline, the physical exertion temporarily took me away from the constant pressure of pre-mature adulthood. Home matches were cheap, as in "free", entertainment. Away matches gave us a chance to visit our families.

During a wrestling match against MIT, I went for a double leg take down and my opponent's reflex drove his knee into my nose. Result: an impact that left stars in my eyes and blood on the mat. Two days later, my nasal cartilage became curved like the letter "C" and I developed a large nasal hematoma. The coach arranged for an ENT consult in Northhampton, seven miles away.

It was dead winter, mid-February and snowing heavily. We had no snow tires so I knew it would be tough sledding. Five miles on Route 7 and the car started to overheat. Steam billowed from under the hood and fogged the windshield. Blinded, I pulled over and into the snow bank. Swearing softly, I stomped around to the front of the car and raised the hood and quickly disappeared in the cloud of steam coming from the engine.

Where was Opa when I needed him?

Without thinking I grasped the radiator cap and promptly burned my hand. Grabbing a towel from the car, I returned to the engine and—-yes, unscrewed the cap—-the blast of hyper-heated radiator fluid pushed me backwards onto the highway flat on my back. I watched in horror as a large delivery truck swerved at the last moment before it would have flattened my skull onto the pavement. My whole head felt like it was on fire, and I managed to roll to the side of the road to sit in the snow bank. Grabbing handfuls of the loose snow, brushing off the grit covering it, I held the clean, cold snow onto my face. It melted quickly, sending rivulets of water down the sides of my hands and into the sleeves of my jacket. A police car drove by, picked me up and transported me to Cooley Dickenson Hospital, my face buried in my snow-filled gloves. Upon arriving at the ER, my face was so swollen that my nasal injury was secondary. Fortunately the burns on my face and scalp were only first and minor second degree even though I looked like the inside of an overripe watermelon covered with Neosporin ointment. And, oh yes, I have a deviated septum to this day.

Six months later I graduated from Amherst. It was not the emotionally explosive event I had anticipated, not at all like the West Point cadets who throw their caps high into the air and let out a hearty "hoorah"! In a word, it was anticlimactic. I had a wife, a 9 month-old baby daughter and years of education, very expensive medical education, ahead of me. That's what I had on my mind.

My dad, a man of few words and stoic demeanor, put out his hand and gave me his time-honored expression of approval, "Way to go, Butch". Why he called me Butch I'll never know. I never asked him, nor did anyone else in the family. I just know that when he was upset I was "Richard", for every day address I was "Rich", and for moments of greetings, good-bye's or kudos, I was "Butch". But that was enough. I know he loved me, though he never, ever said it. He guided me with his love, tough love as it was; and I thirsted and strove for his approval my entire life. He always kept that carrot just barely beyond my reach. It works for some people, and I guess it worked for me, though not without a price.

After spending the last eight summers working a range of grunt and inglorious jobs, I decided to elevate my status and tip-toe into the academic realm. Through a connection with my prep school headmaster, Appleton Seaverns, I applied for a teaching job in math at Cardigan Mountain School in Canaan, New Hampshire, located near Dartmouth College. Ap had been not only a shining star of inspiration for me, a mentor in the most elevated sense, but in many ways a father figure, perhaps even a father. He was the nitro fuel in my tank, the after-burner of energy to excel. So when Ap suggested I contact Mr. John Browning, Assistant Headmaster at the Cardigan School, I did so pronto, with full expectation that I had a good shot at the job. That was in March, three months before graduation. Mr. Browning wanted to meet me. I told him I was on the rugby team and Amherst was playing Dartmouth in two weeks. Well, we beat the pants off Dartmouth—Amherst in our purple and white striped rugby shirts; Dartmouth in theirs—green and white. It was a beautiful, crisp spring day, the kind of day my parents taught me to be thankful for. The playing field was soft from a recent rain and by game's end our uniforms had turned grass green and mud brown, with clogs of sod on our shirts and in our cleats. I met Mr. Browning next to the traditional game's end keg of beer.

"Richard? Richard German?" he asked.

"Mr. Browning?" I asked.

"Yes" we both said together.

He put out his hand and insisted on grasping my grass-stained, dirt caked claw before I could wipe it off. That was my interview, and by the time we finished our beer, he said, "We'll see you at Cardigan in June."

"Thank you, sir, I look forward to it."

I guess that meant I was accepted.

A week after graduation, Carol, Lynn and I packed into the car, said our good-byes to family and headed for the northern woods of New Hampshire. I taught math and canoeing. My qualification for math was that I had made it though the calculus-physics course at Amherst, and for canoeing was that I had spent many a summer maneuvering our beat-up canoe up the creek in Madison at high tide without flipping it over. Carol worked in the mailroom distributing mail and snacks during the 10 a.m. recess, and started an extra-curricular Drama Club for the students, a very big hit on campus.

My students were by and large a good group of boys (it was an all boys prep school), but they had trouble with geometry and looked bored and glassy-eyed when I got to the section on triangles. Solution: I held class outside, and asked them to calculate the hypotenuse of a right triangle formed by the shadow of an 80 foot tall pine tree. They measured the length of the shadow, added the square of that length to the square of the 80 foot tall tree and took the square root of that sum. Bingo! They now knew Pythagorean Theorem, and they probably know it to this day.

Carol, Lynn and I rambled through the thickets during free moments, and picked fresh-as-you-can-get New Hampshire blueberries, warmed by the sun and dripping with goodness. We returned to the campus with blue tongues and fingers so everyone knew what we were up to. What a kick! Good people and evening cookouts—it was a great summer and a neat way to make some bucks before med school.

We returned to Taunton in late August and made plans for the move to Rochester. I had picked out a small, two bedroom apartment from a Rochester newspaper that the admissions secretary had sent me. The method of selection, sight unseen, was easy—it was affordable, very affordable. Moving day came. I had everything carefully mapped out and calculated. I would pick up the moving van at 8 a.m. Friday in Hartford with my brother-in-law Bill Dobbs, drive to Middletown and load it up with pots, pans, bed, crib, hand-me-down and somewhat dented furniture, books, radio (no TV.) and clothes, then drive at breakneck speed to Rochester, unload and carry all that crap up 23 cement steps to the apartment above a furniture store on Chili Avenue, and drive all the way back to Hartford by 7:59 a.m. Saturday to avoid exceeding the 24 hour rental charge. Which we did by 22 minutes! God bless my brother-in-law.

I got a quick 4 hours of sleep and the three of us left for Rochester—our new home for the next 6 years. And what a 6 years it turned out to be!

CHAPTER FOUR

FIRST DAY, FIRST YEAR

*"Go confidently in the direction
of your dreams."*
Henry David Thoreau, American author

"Easier Said Than Done",
The Essex, 1963

September 1963.

"Welcome to the class of '67." The be-speckled, balding man with eyes so pale he didn't seem to have pupils, peered at the classroom filled with first year med students. "I am Dr. Rubin, Professor of Anatomy."

My classmates stared at the podium as we focused on every word coming from the professor's thin-lipped mouth. Somewhat intimidated by the prospect of the next four years, we sat there wide-eyed and stone silent.

"In four years most of you will become doctors," Dr. Rubin risked the flash of a humorless smile. "I say 'most' because statistically a few of you will drop out for various reasons—probably two or three out of this class of 72 students."

Only 2 or 3 of us won't graduate? I thought. *Not bad odds for me to finish…*

"So my advice is, if you are in a relationship, don't get married!" Dr. Rubin's voice rose in emphasis.

I'm already married.

"If you are married," he lowered his eyes to his notes. "Put off having children for a while——say 4 or more years."

Lynn, my 13 month old daughter?

No time to panic.

Too late anyway.

"At precisely 8 a.m. tomorrow," he cleared his throat and fiddled with his bow tie as if he were strangled by it. "You will be assigned a cadaver."

"You are one student in a group of four."

"You will be with your cadaver every day for the next 8 months."

"You will become familiar with your cadaver's every organ, nerve, vessel, bifurcation(Y-shaped division of an artery), muscle, tendon and bone."

"Your anatomy book is your Bible—eat with it, go to sleep with it, take it to the bathroom—in short, commit it to memory." With his thumb, he pushed his glasses up on his nose, and then returned to his notes. We knew this was an affectation since he had delivered this speech on the first Monday of September for the past 15 years. "Here, at the University of Rochester, we demand rapid, accurate recall. Anything less is unacceptable."

He paused dramatically and surveyed the room with colorless eyes.

".... And you will know how it fits together, every bone, every muscle, every cell."

Another unnecessary glance at his notes in order to let his last statement sink in. "You will smell like formaldehyde."

"Use only the morgue elevator at the back of the hospital." He peered over his reading glasses that have already slipped back to the tip of his narrow nose. "Never walk onto the clinical floors, never use the patient elevators...and <u>never, ever</u> enter this facility by the main entrance. Do I make myself clear?"

Pausing, perhaps awaiting a reaction and when there was none, he continued, "Please proceed to the storage room and transport your cadaver down to the dissecting lab..."

I was one of 4 men in our group, lucky number 11. My cadaver partners were white Anglo Saxon males as there were very few females admitted to medical schools in the early 1960's. There were only five women in our class of seventy-two. These were the men with whom I would spend more time than my wife and family in the upcoming year. These were the men with whom I'd partner, compete, and carve up a human being ...

At the time, I had not considered the reality of medical school: a grueling 4 year journey, a gauntlet of 48 nonstop months of work, 1000 hours of class and lab time, 1000 hours of clinical time with patients, 1200 hours of study time and 300 total hours of exam taking. That translates into a lot of energy.

More than that, it is a testament to the very human element of perseverance. This one trait far outshines nearly every other asset: faith, hope, good looks, intellect, money and personality all pale in comparison to the single most significant ingredient, determination: setting a goal, forging through thick and thin, ignoring distractions no matter how tempting, and absolutely staying on track until the goal is achieved, even if not to absolute perfection.

It is the journey rather than the destination that indicates who you are at your core; not the achievement itself, nor the perfection applied along the way. The journey is the true measure of the standards one sets for oneself. The MD degree is the golden gift at the end of the rainbow.

Toby looked barely old enough to shave. With a thatch of blond curly hair, and a florid round face, he gave the impression of carrying too much weight beneath his harsh white lab coat. Adding to that a soft tidewater accent behind a broad toothy smile, Toby might have trouble instilling confidence in his future patients, unless they were all children.

Frank's slight build indicated a hyper-thyroid metabolism. His pale face looked like he had lived in a cave since birth. Male pattern baldness had already removed a considerable amount of his hair for a man still in his early twenties. The large Buddy Holly glasses exaggerated the brown eyes behind them. If clichés could walk or talk, Frank's "nerd" genius appearance almost guaranteed his good performance.

A quick glance at Bill whose deep tan indicated a summer spent on the golf course, and Bass Weejun loafers indicated he could afford it. Sharply creased cashmere slacks, and a well starched Abercrombie button down shirt, completed the picture of a preppie. A trace of toilet paper clung to the spot where he had cut himself shaving a few hours ago. Perhaps he'll go into psychiatry...or anything else not requiring manual dexterity.

"Walk Right In",
The Rooftop Singers, 1963

After cursory introductions, handshakes, nervous smiles and nods, we made our way to the cadaver storage room. True to Dr. Rubin's speech, I smelled the formaldehyde through the solid grey metal door at the end of the hallway. The handle was cold when I jerked the door open and stepped inside. What greeted me made me suddenly stop. I sensed my lab partners piling into each other behind me when they saw the contents of this room.

"Oh, my God…" Toby's soft voice in shock or reverence—-it was hard to tell which.

"Jeez," Bill's clipped Connecticut accent.

Silence from Frank.

"Ahhh…." fell from my open mouth.

Dozens of cadavers all wrapped, mummified-style, in strips of tan cloth were vertically suspended by heavy tongs inserted into the ear canals (the petrous bone is one of the strongest and densest bones in the human body). Hanging from an overhead rack—one after the other after the other—-they looked queued up as if waiting for the latest version of the iPhone. A very efficient, space conserving method of storing bodies, the visual impact was powerful, taking my breath away, followed seconds later by a sudden stinging in my eyes and nose from the pungent chemical effect of cold formalin.

"Aaargh," covering my mouth with my hand I backed into one of my lab partners behind me. He in turn backed into another one, until the one bringing up the rear plunged through the heavy door behind us, releasing us into the hallway.

Stumbling over each other, wiping our eyes, recovering our composure, we glanced around the group and laughed nervously.

"Paper, scissors, rock?" I asked, referring to the kid's game of deciding who gets to go first.

Toby laughed, Bill grunted, and Frank was silent in apparent confusion about what I was referring to.

"Hup, Hup, Ho." Toby, Bill and Rich shook their hands in the circle as Frank opened the door, returning to the room to claim our cadaver.

Welcome to medical school.

CHAPTER FIVE

HARBOR/HAVEN

"A ship is safe in harbor,
but that's not what ships are for"
William Shedd, *author*

"Red Sails in the Sunset",
Fats Domino, 1963

During our first four years in Rochester, we rented a two bedroom apartment, small and old, but adequate. Located 23 cement steps above a furniture store on the main drag, we heard street noises 24/7. Horns, backfires, intermittent yelling, an occasional scream or two, and loud conversations peppered with short, yet to the point, accusations and unflattering descriptions of someone's mother.

There were two adjacent apartments; one housed a single mom and her 9 year-old son, the other, an older couple who argued sporadically. We overlooked a garage in the rear next to the dumpster. Rent was $65 a month, plus another $5 for the fridge. However, the landlord agreed to take $5 off if I collected the garbage twice a week for the entire apartment complex. So my part time job was that of a trash collector—once again. Carol worked as assistant to the buyer for ladies dresses in a large department store. We managed to survive...survival being the operative word.

Expenses were minimized. Being a frugal Yankee, I bought used books whenever I could. Histology (the study of normal tissue) required a microscope, so I bought a third-hand monocular for $50 from a senior med student and wore an eye patch so I wouldn't have to squint. At exam time, I borrowed a Zeiss binocular microscope with zoom lens from Bill, my buddy, and dumped the eye patch. We worked together painting houses during the summer, so it all worked out.

Carol and I had a routine that kept our heads above water. Lynn was a great kid, a real sleeper, and our design was to keep her up late (probably known as child abuse today) while I studied, then we all collapsed for a good night's sleep around midnight. Lynn would wake up around 6AM, and the day started. Carol fed Lynn, but the thought of facing my cadaver, soaked in formalin, festered deep in my stomach and removed all desire to ingest any measure of breakfast. In fact, I got out of the habit of eating breakfast for the next 4 years, and only during the food deprivation of internship did I return to gobbling down a donut and some OJ on the way up to the OR.

Carol packed Lynn up for the baby sitter and left by 8AM, making it to work at Sibley, Lindsey & Curr in downtown Rochester by 9AM. The baby sitter, 35 year old Grace, and her husband Frank who worked for Delco Battery, were two of God's angels. They lived 5 minutes from our apartment in a modest, compact two story, grey shingled Archie Bunker-type house with 5 kids, 3 of their own and 2 "adopted" from single moms who slowly faded away leaving their children for Grace and Frank to raise. It reminded me of the "old woman in the shoe" house, which had the magical ability to accommodate the needs of the many children she cared for, which totaled at least 13 during the day. These kids were entertained, happy and ever so gently disciplined. Within the confines of the chain-link fenced-in back yard for hours at a time, children of all ages played games, ran around and generally had a good time. In the winter, this magic moved indoors. How Grace managed to potty-train, feed, nose wipe, care for, love and yes, even adopt, these children was a gift from heaven that I never saw in another human being, ever. And, like my own sister, Gracie always had time to hug me hello and goodbye with her skinny arms. To this day I close my eyes and can see her sparkling eyes and beaming smile. What a woman!

If Carol and I could coordinate, she would drive me to the hospital 15 minutes away. Otherwise I pumped my own way on a second-hand bicycle, the tires half-eaten by Rochester's winter salt.

Anatomy class started at 8:30 AM sharp, "not 8:31 AM" as Dr. Rubin had warned. Three and one-half hours of sifting through Jonas, with no breakfast aboard, definitely left me hungry for lunch. The students and house staff had a separate dining hall, and it literally hummed with vibrancy in between and even during bites of hospital food. At 1PM we assembled, all 72 of us, in the grand Whipple Auditorium, named for our pathology professor and director of the medical school, George Hoyt Whipple, M.D., who had received the Nobel Prize in Medicine in 1934 for his discovery of pernicious anemia. He was a giant of a man. He loved to keep his shot-gun on the book shelf, at the ready for an occasional pheasant that might wander out of the near-by woods and past his office. Here in this hall of revered voices, we endured the mundane drone of our histology professor, a most somnolent experience indeed. One learned how to appear to be taking notes while in a semi-sleep zone, a talent I transferred to the operating table years later as an exhausted intern where I learned how to hold a Deaver retractor and semi-sleep at the same time. The next 2 hours, most of us retired to the library and caught up on some serious study in preparation for the next day, be it an exam or a new chapter. At 5:30 PM, 6 of us would beat it down to the gym and play some 3-on-3 hoops for a wild hour of physical release. A quick shower and I was home for supper where Carol, God bless her, had put in 8 hours of work, earned the bacon, picked up Lynn and always provided a creative meal, albeit within our modest budget. Then back to 4 more hours of study before that blessed event I called sleep.

CHAPTER SIX

BODY AND SOUL

*"It's always darkest
before it's totally black".*
Charlie Brown, "Peanuts"

"I'm on the Outside Looking In",
Little Anthony & The Imperials, 1966

Each cadaver was identified by a number attached to the wrist.

"What was that number again?" I snapped at Frank who held our assignment number a few inches from his bespectacled eyes.

"29, damnit!" He snapped back.

"Am I looking for a male or a female?" I asked, my voice betraying my ambivalence surrounding what we were about to do.

"How the hell should I know?" Frank responded.

I heard a chortle from Toby who was bringing up the rear. "Hey, Yankee, look for some lipstick—Southern women never go anywhere without it."

"Gentlemen, please, a little respect among the dead," Bill's clipped Connecticut accent did not hide the sarcasm behind his remark.

I remembered a classics professor at Amherst when he referred to users of sarcasm as "fearful beings tearing at their own flesh."

All too soon, we would all be tearing someone else's flesh.

The higher the number the deeper one had to wander into the storage room to find the matching cadaver. Someone's teeth were chattering behind me. Bumping our way between swinging bodies, rubbing our stinging eyes and snuffling driblets of formalin, we finally found our man. I was the designated hitter, so I shoved the hanging cadaver with my hand in the middle of his back and pushed him toward the door as his body traveled along the overhead pulley, like a side of beef in a freezer. All four of us lifted him loose from the hook, and then lowered him from the pulley, gently placing him on the metal gurney, stiffer than a frozen tuna and seemed to be twice as heavy.

After only two minutes of exposure to this chemical fog, we smelled worse than the cadaver. And a shower was twelve hours away.

"Should we name him?" asked Bill.

"How about Jonas?" contributed Toby, in his soft Southern drawl.

"What does the stiff have to do with a whale?" Bill asked.

"Not Jonah, moron. Joan-ASS, as in Salk," Frank's voice dripped with condescension.

I flipped his tag to check what his real name was, but all I saw was his number, 29 and the date. "No help here."

"Ok, Jonas, it is..." Bill ended the discussion before hacking and coughing in a futile attempt to clear the smell from his nose, and the taste from his mouth.

Like pallbearers, two of us on either side of the aluminum gurney, we marched in time toward the morgue elevator en route to the dissection room two floors above. During the 20 second elevator trip, stone silence surrounding us, I could feel my heart pounding, my eyes stinging as I tried to display the confidence of a real doctor. I glanced at my three partners in cadaver dissection. Toby's blue eyes seemed glued to the ceiling, Frank's bulging brown eyes stared at his shoes, and Bill's eyes were closed.

Sucking in my stomach, straightening my spine, I renewed my determination to ace anatomy. Suddenly I was in the big leagues—no more purple mouse kidney tissue smeared onto a slide, no more frog dissections in undergraduate biology 101, and the cat...I don't like to think about the cat. Tentatively, my index finger touched the thick tan cotton canvas wrapped around Jonas the cadaver, our cadaver, my cadaver. This was the real thing: a body belonging to somebody's brother, somebody's father, somebody's son...now a piece of meat destined for dissection, a learning experience for ambitious medical students. Formerly an efficient machine with moveable parts, functioning organs, and a level of intelligence generous enough to donate his body to a bunch of medical students eager to learn. Ninety percent of cadavers used by medical schools are unclaimed bodies, ten percent are donated pre-mortem. Jonas was now a whole entity soon to be separated into inanimate systems revealing the mystery of his former life.

But not his personality, not his spirit, and not his soul.

Jonas had taken those with him.

Why was I here?

How did I get here?

"Turn, Turn, Turn"
(To Everything There is a Season),
The Byrds, 1965

I owed it to Binky Minor, my best friend. I was 15 and he was 16 years old when we sped along the winding rural roads in his yellow '54 Ford Fairlane convertible. What a hot car—necker's knob (some of us called it a suicide knob, since the driver spun the wheel while he was necking with his girlfriend in the passenger seat) on the steering wheel, glass pack mufflers and a chrome tail pipe extension. Blasting Bill Haley and the Comets' "Rock Around the Clock", top down, warmed by early summer sunshine, enjoying this incredible sense of freedom, we shared our free time, our short term dreams and long term ambitions. His dad was a doctor and of course he would be a doctor, too.

Summer came and we moved to our summer cottage in Madison on Long Island Sound, 25 miles away. Mom told me Binky had developed a lump in his neck; it was called Hodgkin's disease, a new and unfamiliar word for me. His parents had taken him to the Leahy Clinic in Boston for treatment. I looked forward to seeing him in September when we would move back to Middletown for the school year.

The day we left Madison, Mom told me Binky had died. Shocked disbelief at this sudden revelation, I dropped to the floor and cried. Long, moaning ululations, red-faced denial followed by blinding rage as I struggled to my feet and faced my parents.

They stood a few feet apart; my mother looking down at the faded dishtowel in her hands, my father staring at me his mouth slightly open in apparent surprise.

Fists clenched at my side, my face reddened in a rage I didn't think possible, directed at my parents. "Why didn't you tell me?! How could you NOT tell me? Binky is my best friend!"

As if I were Lot, who had just turned his wife to a pillar of salt, I stared at my parents, stiff as stones looking back at me.

Overwhelmed with emotions I had never felt before and didn't know I possessed, I felt any semblance of self control drain from my body. Red hot rage replaced it, forcing me to pace back and forth, back and forth in front of my paralyzed parents.

Wave after wave of grief, anger and frustration swamped me, threatening to drown me in intense feelings of loss, abandonment and anger. Gulping and gasping for air in this suddenly close kitchen, I struggled to express my sense of their betrayal. Shaking my head in disbelief that they had kept this from me....first the severity of his illness, then his death.

Didn't they trust me enough to tell me, or didn't they think I was mature enough to deal with it, or didn't they know me well enough to realize that Binky and I were very best friends? I had not known the reality of any of it —-preventing me from saying good-by to my very best friend.

To this day, I wonder if Binky forgave me for not seeing him, for not being there for him, for not acting like his very best friend when he needed me the most.

The day he died the world lost a young man destined to be a highly skilled physician.

The day he died was the day I decided to become a doctor.

Deciding to become a surgeon came later...much later.

Med students are the same as any other graduate level group. Their personalities are a cross-section of all types— some aggressive, with a short- term gratification fuse who are destined to become surgeons; some reflective and more gentle souls who gravitate into more delayed gratification roles like psychiatry, internal medicine and neurology; there are others who are not "people" people and prefer the isolation and independence of the laboratory, either as a pathologist or researcher.

Our dissecting group had four diverse and distinct personalities. To my surprise, soft spoken Toby from the Tidewater area of Virginia, was our resident intellect. He excelled in all subjects requiring extensively detailed instant recall, especially the basic sciences. Having been accepted to both law and medical school, he opted for the latter. High energy and a quick study, Toby seemed in motion even when he stood still, keeping his own counsel as he studied the open abdomen of a freshly incised cadaver. His fleshy face gave no hint of the muscular body beneath the starched white lab coat. Friendly, as only Virginians can be, his infectious laugh accompanied a well-timed zinger which lightened the tension in the room.

Frank's bulging brown eyes behind thick lenses saw things that the rest of us missed. It wasn't the magnification of the glasses that gave him laser like vision, it was that large brain beneath his prematurely balding pate that managed to stay one or two steps ahead of the rest of us. Often he provided answers before the question was asked, a habit that disconcerted more than one of our professors. Cerebral Frank was a soft spoken violin virtuoso who often indulged in reading Plato in the original Latin when he was not stuck in the porta hepatus. The rest of us wondered why he selected medical school instead of Juilliard or Peabody for his post graduate studies. My guess was that having mastered music, this was another frontier for his insatiable intellect.

Beneath the Brooks Brothers clothing Bill was as big as an ex-football player from an Ivy League school could be—-average size American male. Boisterous and good hearted with a deep guttural laugh and an appetite that transcended the reasonable, Bill always brought a brown bag for a mid-morning meal to keep his inefficient metabolism fueled. Standing back from the cadaver, he wiped his fingers on his lab coat (we wore no gloves in anatomy) before diving into a meatloaf sandwich, leaving greasy fingerprints on the white bread in between bites.

Frank's repulsion was indicated when his mouth fell open in shock the first time Bill ate one of his many snacks standing next to Jonas. One day during dissection of the intestines, Bill came in early and lined the cadaver's open abdominal cavity with saran wrap and dumped in a bowl of homemade beef stew. In came Frank, and there was Bill holding his anatomy book in his left hand and with his right hand eating beef stew with a huge long spoon from the cadaver's abdomen. Apparently aware of Frank's presence, Bill with stew dribbling down his chin, looked up and grinned at Frank who damn near threw up on the spot.

This was 18 years before AIDS was identified, and we were given absolutely no information regarding any possible transmittable diseases (hepatitis, T.B., etc.) regarding our cadaver. We all assumed, probably correctly, that the pathology department had screened all deceased bodies before allowing them to become candidates for cadaver dissection. Since we did not wear gloves, our fingertips became wrinkled under the influence of 8 hours of formalin exposure each day, our fingernails a repository for bits of unsavory anatomy which we assiduously washed away at day's end. The perfume of formalin lingered like the juice of wild Connecticut skunk cabbage we had rolled in as kids, much to my parents' displeasure. Some things never change. My father's admonition, "Richard, you stink—go wash up" simply morphed into Carol's patient suggestion, "Rich honey, why don't you relax in a hot tub while I make dinner!"

Near the end of anatomy course, prior to the important final exam, we had two final areas to dissect, the pelvis and the brain. The female pelvis is somewhat difficult to approach since the cadaver legs are frozen in extension and must be flexed at the hips into the lithotomy position (as if to deliver a baby, or have a pelvic exam). The legs are held up and apart by an inverted U-shaped bar which is attached to the end of the dissecting table. First, one must slide the cadaver down so her buttocks are at the very end of the table, at which point the hips are forcibly flexed upward so the legs can be attached to the overhead bar.

Four med students adjacent to our table got as far as sliding their female cadaver to the end of the table. The cadaver, however, kept sliding...and sliding until she slid completely off the slick, Vaseline greased stainless steel table taking all four med students down to the floor, corpse and all. In stunned silence, the rest of us rushed from our seats, falling all over each other to assist in the recovery effort. From the expression on his face, this was a first for Dr. Rubin as his glasses remained where they belonged, on the bridge of his nose.

The following day, our entire class had assembled in the auditorium to observe the professor in his dissection of the pelvis. His assistant rolled in a metal gurney with a two foot long object covered by a white sheet. He removed the sheet. There was a female torso, transected above at the level of the pubic bone and below across both thighs, a segment of what had previously been a woman. He used a long probe that he inserted down into the transected specimen, pointing out the ovaries, fimbriated fallopian tubes, suspensory ligaments, uterus and so on. I couldn't imagine what had happened to that young woman whose truncated pelvic torso was now being probed and prodded in great depth and detail.

I felt the recent cup of coffee and gut bomb rising in the back of my throat. Afraid to risk a glance at Toby or Bill, sitting on either side of me, I swallowed hard forcing the poor excuse for a breakfast back down. I heard other people fake coughing around me, probably trying to resist the urge most of us felt: blowing chunks all over our shoes.

After seven months of dissecting the human body, very little affected us. But I witness that scene to this day....the impact I felt then remains in force today.

As Dr. Rubin had explained a few short months ago, the mysterious and confusing would transition to the recognizable and understandable as we slowly coalesced all of the disparate information into a cohesive, interrelated anatomic structure called the human body. The final frontier, the human brain, was reserved for the end of the course.

We made a large U-shaped incision through the skin of entire scalp and pulled it completely back. We then cut through the skull with an oscillating circular saw and removed the bony cap to reveal the thick, protective grey dura covering the brain. After cutting away the dura, there rested the brain in all its glory, road mapped by tiny blue-gray veins containing stagnant dark blood coursing along its surface and valleys.

Yes, this was another part of the cadaver and by now we were fairly hardened to the fact it had once been a living, breathing human being who had become an inanimate piece of meat. However, in spite of my best intentions, my thoughts went to questions about what experiences, ideas, realizations, feelings and emotions had passed through this tissue weighing down my hand.

CHAPTER SEVEN

THE HUMAN MACHINE: A DIVINE DESIGN

"Man has made many machines, complex and cunning, but which of them indeed rivals the workings of the heart"
Pablo Casals, cellist and conductor

"Venus",
Frankie Avalon, 1960

First year med school is the study of the body's normal condition: anatomy, physiology(the workings of an organ), histology(microscopic study of body/organ cells) and hematology(blood cells of all types, and there are a bunch), the language of the human body, the required courses that make up a medical degree. As in most sciences, it helped to establish the parameters of normalcy before venturing into the realm of abnormal.

By the end of the year, anatomy had taught us the normal structure of the human body, literally from the head to the toe. There comes a time beyond which one cannot learn without some hands-on experience. Hence, Jonas and his evil twin, Judith, the corpse with Revlon's "Fire and Ice" chipped nail polish on her cold dead hand on the adjacent table.

We had grown quite attached to our cadavers. By the end of the eight month course, Jonas had little resemblance to the individual who had donated his body. Rather he looked more and more like all the rest of them, stripped of personality, individuality, and distinction. We had completely shredded, sliced and probed each part of them. Jonas, Judith and their lifeless associates were indistinguishable from each other. At the end of the course, they looked like leftover spaghetti.

We had removed the brain during dissection leaving the empty skull a cavernous hole. In order to separate the spinal column posteriorly from the esophagus anteriorly, we had sawed the bone straight down from the top of the head to behind the ears. The top of the skull, like half of a coconut shell, held the two portions together. When the restraining skull cap had been removed, it flopped apart in a rather macabre fashion. In the immortal words of William Shakespeare's character Falstaff, "Alas, poor Yorrick, I knew him ..."

Physiology, the study of how organs function—how the heart pumps, muscles contract, kidneys filter, liver detoxifies and the lungs exchange gases was one of the more exciting and fascinating disciplines in medical school. The "how" of things has always appealed to me, and I spent a lot of time figuring out how an engine produced power, a radio received and transmitted signals, and how a bumblebee survives when it's technically too heavy to fly.

If it moved, I was interested.

Physiology increased my interest in surgery. Each organ has its separate purpose contributing to the effective functioning of the whole human being. Structurally perfect, efficient, and one of the wonders of nature, our organs are engineering miracles. Perhaps it was genetic, Opa's influence on my DNA that made machinery an object of fascination for me. Converting material into fuel and fuel into energy and energy into action is a process that continuously propels progress, both environmental and evolutionary. .

The argument can be made that technologic evolution has made many engineering innovations obsolete. In its time, the steam locomotive and internal combustion engine replaced the horse drawn wagons and carriages. Ship power plants evolved from sail to steam to oil to nuclear power. Each advance contains the seeds of its own destruction. Medicine evolved from "biting the bullet" to sophisticated localized and general anesthetics, from Civil War leg amputations aided by a swig of whiskey (for patient and doctor) to current day surgery.

In terms of the human body, surgeons regularly remove tonsils, adenoids and appendixes which have malfunctioned and are no longer necessary to the functioning of the machine. Almost without realizing it, I became focused on the surgery option in medicine. To remove or repair parts of the living, breathing person seemed a natural outlet for my focus on how things work, what they feel like, and a manual dexterity probably inherited from Opa.

Therefore histology, the study of microscopic appearance of normal tissue, put me to sleep even thinking about it. The classes started just after lunch at 1:00 p.m. and lasted two and one-half hours in a stuffy over-heated lecture hall. At 1:05 p.m., the professor turned off the lights in Whipple Auditorium, and the professor's soft monotone quickly assumed white noise proportions as he described each organ's normalcy. One by one, heads nodded, eyes closed, breathing deepened and each of us slowly but surely drifted off to sleep. The course was notorious for its universal soporific effect.

Suddenly a full color, 6' X 6' Miss February centerfold filled the pull down screen and jolted us out of repose, the professor's idea of Haydn's "Surprise Symphony".

Just as quickly, the centerfold was gone.

Damn! I should have stayed awake. Sex always works!

CHAPTER EIGHT

THE FINAL EXAM

"There is no end to education.
It is not that you read a book,
pass an examination... The whole of life...
is a process of learning"
Jiddu Krishnamurti, Indian philosopher

"Don't know much about history, don't
know much biology. . ."
"What a Wonderful World This Would Be",
Sam Cooke, 1960

Outside the tall slender windows of the dissection
room, night had fallen hours earlier. Yellow lights from
the high ceiling illuminated Jonas, my dormant anatomy
instructor now that my team members had retired for the
night. Only a few of us remained to study for the Anatomy
final early tomorrow morning.

Quiet, like a linen shroud, enveloped us. Scratchy,
thick and oppressive, the garment wrapped us in solitude
and mental exhaustion. Our future depended on our performance in a few short hours, and yet that future seemed
forever away. Shaking my head to return my attention to
Jonas who contained the answers to all of the questions on
tomorrow's exam, I snapped back into focus...sort of.

My stomach rumbled.

A headache started behind my eyes.

The effort it took not to yawn drew my attention from my text book to the naked clock staring at me from the darkened wall over my left shoulder.

Tuesday, 10:30 p.m.

I had the mediastinum(the space between the lungs, rich with various structures and lymph nodes), lungs and heart left to review for the anatomy exam.

And I hadn't eaten in over 8 hours.

And my first anatomy exam was a little over 8 hours away.

And my family?

The musky odor of the cadaver's viscera, mingled with the sharp pungency of the formalin soaked tissue, periodically stung my eyes and nose. My attention shifted from any serious thoughts of food. Resignation came from a glance around the room reconfirming the presence of a few other med students hunched over their cadavers. Their backs aching like mine, their eyes bloodshot from the strain, their minds numb from the onslaught of detailed information.

The soft background whir of an overburdened fan and the abrupt snap of a page someone turned in their anatomy book were the only sounds. The sharpness of the intermittent interruptions was somewhat disturbing leaning toward annoying, like a hacking cough barking when you are trying to nap.

The pages of my used anatomy book had been softened by my predecessors who had taken this same anatomy course every year for the past decade. They contained the greasy thumb and fingerprints of hands that had invaded every cavity, every lumen (the inside of any hollow structure, ie intestine, colon, blood vessels, etc), and every organ in the body.

We were way past modesty in this liaison which pitted my physical, mental and emotional endurance against that inert conglomeration of tissue which had been systematically invaded by my unskilled hands holding inanimate instruments. We were an odiferous unit, my cadaver, my book and I. We stank together, toiled together and passed through emotional phases together.

As I sat on my tall hard wooden stool, Jonas—-or what was left of Jonas—-stretched out in repose before me. Remembering the first time I saw Jonas unzipped and exposed to the naïve eyes, eager minds, and frozen emotions of our team, I recalled how difficult my first few weeks of anatomy had been.

Not the work so much as my effort to overcome my subjective involvement with that former human being lying in front of me. I could not repress thoughts of what he might have been like, what his life was about, who loved him, who did he love and leave, was he in pain at the moment of death; if so, what from and what he was doing while I was a high school student or water skiing on Long Island Sound in the summer.

What incredible series of circumstances brought the two of us together in this unusual association; now we were involved in a very intimate, one-way relationship. I was gaining valuable information thanks to his generosity, and his body was the sacrifice. My knife blade would separate tissues, but give no pain. His unchanging catatonic face betrayed no response to my persistent manipulations, investigative intrusions, or deep probing.

Judith, the other students' cadaver, was female with fingernails still showing specks of bright red nail polish. After a glance at her, I often wondered what she had thought and where she was sitting when that polish was applied for the last time.

Another cadaver was a young man...a teenager. What biologic catastrophe had occurred inside him for his body to end up here on a cold steel table teaching med students what they needed to know before applying that knowledge to people with a pulse?

In a sense, he still existed lying motionless on the slippery, gleaming metallic table in tangible organic form. As much as any inert group of molecules exist, he was present in this reality, in our reality. Yet, where was that complex ingredient that once made him kinetic? Where was the plug that made him fun? In this sense, death did not seem such a radical departure from life. No mystical metamorphosis had occurred. His body was in front of me as it once had been in front of a mirror shaving. Death had denied the biologic coincidence of function and the ability to realize its existence. I thought back to Nat Turner, the angry and frustrated black man who, in the darkness of the plantation era in Colonial America that brutalized so many slaves, rounded up twelve of his enslaved fellow men and slaughtered the white inhabitants of several households. One of his victims, butchered by Nat's machete, was described as having been dragged down the grand wooden staircase by the feet, the murdered man's head bouncing from stair to stair, obeying only the laws of physics in the absence of any physiologic response. Devoid of all life, the repetitive "thump, thump, thump" of his head against each step was all that remained.

If the others in my group had experienced the thoughts that haunted me intensely during my early months of study, they didn't admit it. For the first time I came to look at death as the culmination of denials and was frustrated by the absolute predestination of it all. It bothered me that I had no control over these morbid thoughts which culminated into two horrible nightmares.

The first occurred in October, a month after I had started med school. My Jonas, our cadaver, completely shredded by my thorough efforts of dissection over the past weeks of anatomy lab, somehow had awakened from the sort-of coma he had apparently been in. He struggled to sit up from the dissecting table, and then feet first, he slid onto the floor. Jonas was only dangling cloth and shredded anatomy, standing quietly and communicating, by his catatonic stare, the tragedy of the situation. Drained and dissected, Jonas, the man, could not survive in the bits and pieces in which he now found himself. It was I who had denied him the precious gift of life. Having somehow quietly survived the months of my dissection, now that I was done, Jonas must die—as in the Kafka story, "The Guard" who was tasked with preserving another's life only to die at his post in the end. No one had passed through his gate during his lifetime, a macabre paradox.

I awoke with a start, and remembered the dream in great detail. I thought of Mary, the girl in "Our Town" by Thornton Wilder, who spoke through her own death of the preciousness of life.

My parents, especially Mom, taught me a great reverence for life, and I grew up as a very tactile young boy. I

loved to smell all varieties of fragrances: roses in our garden, fresh baked bread in the oven, Mom's perfume, dad's
linseed oil for his paint brushes, freshly cut rhubarb from
the back yard by the willow tree. To this day the smell of a
mowed lawn transports me instantly to my pleasant chores
as a young boy and how proud I was to show Dad how well
I had cut the grass. And I loved the texture of things- my
dog's furry back, the butter smooth hand made maple dining room table, the back of a Japanese beetle that fed off
the roses, and the oiled feathers of our sky blue pet para-
keet. I was not about to miss these pleasures of life that
Mary had been so tragically denied.

Two months later, the second dream found me in a
rundown attic portion of the hospital. The room had been
converted into a terminal ward. Every patient had a biologic time bomb which systematically erased one life after
the other in sporadic though predictable fashion. The
patients were very old and very ill. Evidently I had been
there to try and comfort them. As I walked by an old
woman's bed, she cried out for me. We both realized her
time to die had arrived and when I reached out to her she
grasped my arm in her tight bony hand as if to drag me
along with her. I struggled frantically to free myself. That
sensation of frantic effort dominated the dream—let her
die, let me live. A plea...

I snapped back into reality. I could not afford emotional diversions while attempting to learn the course of
the vagus nerve. The longest autonomic nerve in the body,
this founding member of the parasympathetic family,
known as the tenth cranial nerve, rises from the base of the
skull in the brain stem and becomes a thick, grayish tube

of nerve fibers that streams down along either side of the esophagus, giving off branches to the larynx and pharynx, then to the heart and lungs. It continues its long descent through an opening in the back of the diaphragm and dissipates into multiple contributory fibers that enervate vessels, intestine and all visceral organs in the abdomen. Finally, terminal branches are sent to the reproductive and urologic organs, all in the service of providing input and balance to the sympathetic family which governs the "fright, fight or flight" response of adrenalin.

"Richard, stop personifying Jonas, and start learning his anatomy," I admonished myself. I stopped fixating on the bright red fingernail polish on the female cadaver across the room, returning my full attention to the liver. Developing detachment is not like flipping the switch on a lamp; it's more like turning down the rheostat on the wall, and the lights gradually dim. Detachment is never an abrupt change; rather it's a gradual process of shifting attention from our emotions to our intellect.

It is not so dramatic as an "Aha!" moment when fluorescent lights suddenly illuminate the sterile field of an operating room and the patient is prepped and ready for surgery; rather it is the evolution of the stoicism developed from hours and hours of sifting around in some cadaver's chest cavity, tracing the course of nerves and blood vessels, missing dinners with my family, canceling the rarely scheduled squash games, and getting used to formalin, bleached fingertips, and stinging eyes.

My cadaver had begun to assume new identities. No longer a "Jonas", he was now an "it", an object for study. It was an opportunity for using surgical instruments; it was a pleasant change from the boredom of bio-chemistry lab; it was always there available, waiting, and silent. An inconvenience to Saturday morning football games, a guilt inducing distraction from time with Lynn and Carol, and a reason for stressful insomnia.

The emotional connotations were gone, dispelled by the phenomenon of conditioning. Hold a hermit crab in your hand and tap on his shell.

He will immediately withdraw. Continue to tap in regular fashion and he will re-emerge despite the disturbance which seconds before initiated the opposite response. So, too, had I been conditioned, though so gradually that the realization hadn't entered my conscious thought?

The unyielding wooden stool beneath my ischial tuberosites (the bones you sit on) put my butt to sleep. The irritating snap of pages jangled me and my neck muscles burned—I wanted to go home and sleep with Carol, I wanted to play with Lynn, mostly I wanted to take a nap; I did not want to sit here and fondle cadaver tissue, or examine nerve pathways, or churn through a worn out anatomy book. Whatever happened to that glorified image of a med student, "savior-in-training", held just a few months before as a college senior?

My team mates lacked the sobering influence of a wife and a child waiting at home for them. Carol and Lynn provided a much needed reality check for me on those rare occasions I found time to spend with them. My team mates were far too private and stoic to discuss such human truths with each other.

Carol was a sympathetic ear and we discussed my existential fantasies and fears in some depth over dinner when the occasion allowed. She offered helpful perspective, though when you feel something so deeply and intensely, it's obviously a real part of your make-up. Time and reality act as a buffer and provide deliverance from the demons. Reality was in the form of a healthy, loving 1 year-old daughter—-her warm, sweet pink vibrancy in stark contrast to the putrid, colorless formalin infused collection of human tissue beneath my dissection blade.

Other medical students released their tension in other ways. Three students from a down state medical school decided to pulled off a prank on the Connecticut-New York Turnpike which, at the time, had toll booths every 30 miles or so. Around midnight, the med students went to the anatomy lab late one night to disarticulate (sever) the left arm of their cadaver at the elbow. They smuggled the human contraband out of the hospital climbed into their car and headed for the turnpike.

The leader sat in the back seat behind the driver, inserted the cadaver arm into his jacket's left sleeve and placed the toll fee, a quarter, in the cadaver hand. He supported the cadaver arm out the window as they approached the toll booth. When the toll collector reached for the quarter, they hit the gas and sped off, leaving the toll collector holding the quarter and half a cadaver arm.

Reports were the toll collector had a heart attack, perhaps a result of the rumor mill. However, why would three presumably intelligent young men risk so much for an unfunny joke? Were they drinking the alcohol used in the process? Had the bizarre juxtaposition of cold grey death and warm colorful life been too much to take for these three med students? Having gone through the academic gauntlet needed for acceptance to med school, how frivolous and wasteful, and then end it all with an incident of such profoundly poor judgment. The three med students were summarily expelled as it was a rather simple task to trace down the only cadaver missing a left forearm. Beyond the demonstration of lack of respect for the person no longer embodied in the cadaver, beyond the effort it took to perform such a ridiculous action, beyond the obvious: perhaps these three did not belong in medicine in the first place. Perhaps they are successful lawyers today.

Each med student had been given a long box containing all the bones of the body at the start of this course. We memorized the names of each and the muscles attached to them, including the origin and insertion (moving end) of muscle. The top of the skull could be lifted off to reveal the twelve foramen (channels in the bone through which nerves passed to reach the face and neck) which had to be studied in detail. I had painstakingly painted twelve broom straws in different colors to represent the corresponding nerves and carefully inserted each straw into its appropriate foramen.

It was 11:00 p.m. the night before the final exam, and my 1 ½ year-old daughter was crawling around by my desk, a pleasant distraction. I got up to get a soda and came back to find that she had just pulled out the twelve straws and was delighted by this bony object that rolled around the floor.

Twelve straws and two hours later, I knew my stuff.

Time for the anatomy exam came—72 students, eighteen cadavers, one big room. Each cadaver had three individually numbered objects to be identified. There were 4 students in a group, 3 minutes per cadaver, then rotating to the next cadaver on instruction from the professor. We had our clipboards and quiz sheet in hand. The anatomy professor asked if there were any questions. This was serious stuff and we were all competing against each other for the best grade.

For the next hour we turned from friends to competitors—dead serious competitors.

The three-minute time clock rang and the exam began.

Ready, set, go.

Is that the recurrent laryngeal or superior thyroid nerve? Shit! . . . Next! That's the celiac axis. I was sure of it . . . Next!

The only thing that overcomes anxiety is knowledge, which can only be achieved by busting one's ass. We all busted our asses, of course, but some did better than others.

Eventually, you learn to work under pressure; if not, go sell insurance. Good-bye. No handholding...just goodbye. Years later, as a surgeon, the pressure tactics pay off. You don't get excited, you don't panic . . . you just intensify, concentrate and persevere and hope like hell your training is instilled in your hands.

CHAPTER NINE

A SUMMER BREAK, SORT OF

"You miss 100% of the shots you never take"
Wayne Gretsky, hockey player

"It's summertime, summertime,
sum, sum, summertime"
"Summertime", The Jamies, 1958

The year was over. I had survived first year of med school. Lynn was nearly two years old, the pervasive smell of formalin was fading, and it was time to re-sell some of my used medical books to the unwary and equally cashed-strapped incoming first-year med student. Clean off the greasy fingerprints and remove bits of cadaver anatomy still stuck to the pages of Tobin's *"Anatomy"* and it looked nearly new—well, almost.

During the school year, Saturday mornings were reserved for family fun. Lynn and I would lie in bed and watch "The Three Stooges" on television for hours. We would laugh and giggle and then go to the Genesee River and picnic with my classmates...weather permitting.

Psych class emphasized the importance of imprinting on young children. So there we lay on our backs in the grass with Lynn sitting on my stomach. An airplane flew overhead, and Freddie, a fellow married med student and good friend, got Lynn's attention, pointed to the airplane and said, "Look, Lynn—a camel, a camel!" So of course

Lynn said, "Camel!", which stuck for awhile. We cracked up.

The summers were a pleasant respite from the grind of medical school. They came abruptly with the warm sun and I had time to put my feet up and laugh. Time for a gin and tonic and Dostoyevsky at 3 o'clock in the afternoon if I wanted. The long afternoons spent on paper chromatography (graphs that show separation of complex mixtures) and serum colorimetry (an instrument used for chemical analysis by comparison of a liquid's color) gained a different perspective with my feet dangling in the swimming pool after a set of tennis...Carol and Lynn waiting for me to appear for a walk, a picnic dinner, or simply taking charge of Lynn so Carol could have some time to herself.

By the end of that first year, I sensed a distance developing between Carol and me...nothing either of us had the time or desire to discuss. Lots of luck with a two year old around every waking moment, and most of those I spent in class, in the lab, or with my nose in a book. Having enough on my plate, I was either unaware of her feelings and therefore unable to do anything about them; or unwilling to add anything else to my already overflowing plate. Probably the latter. Like most men, I pushed any distracting thoughts aside as I focused on what was important to me and my family, Lynn and Carol.

One of the many qualities that attracted me to Carol was her "laissez-faire" approach to life. Almost Zen-like and soothing to the soul, she had the ability to take life as it came in stark contrast to my intensity. Goal oriented, committed to action, and fully aware that the shortest distance between two points was a straight line, I forged ahead with single-minded concentration. At that time in our lives, we complemented each other.

I was a product of my era, chauvinistic as it was. Success oriented, it was my job to provide a future for my family and my priorities took precedence. In retrospect, those societal dictates were already anachronistic. Men were blind to the ambitions of the women in their generation, women were unaware of men's ignorance of their dissatisfaction, and the results played out in the divorce courtrooms across the country.

At that time, Carol and I were unaware of the attitudinal revolution occurring in male/female relationships all around us. Instead, we welcomed the change of routine. My distraction as a summertime house painter provided relief from the mental commitment required in medical school and helped to revive our relationship. Replacing the discipline of mind-numbing, rote learning with the satisfaction of physical exertion allowed Carol back into my life and reminded me why we were together in the first place. At times the focal point of our relationship, and always the third line of our equilateral family triangle, Lynn's presence enriched our lives in so many ways.

My summers were not totally R & R. For me these short weeks meant "Rush for Revenue", and not "Rest and Relaxation". It was my responsibility to play catch-up and earn money to see us through the winter. I had to earn enough money during the summer to pay for the entire year's rent.

Due to my awakening interest in surgery, a staff surgeon invited me to perform my own experiments in the surgical research lab. This eight week fellowship, worth $700, allowed me to operate on rats.

The main frustration in pre-clinical years of med school (first and second years) was the absence of patient contact. Rats weren't exactly patients, but they were living things for which I was expected to take surgical responsibility, and as far as I was concerned this was advanced exposure.

It was exciting to develop a surgical technique for the first time in my life, to be operating in the same lab as the surgical residents and staff surgeons, then to look up the literature pertinent to my experiment. No one gave me direction. It was my own baby. Freedom made all the difference—there was no academic pressure and the work was infinitely more rewarding. Anyhow, I only operated in the lab three mornings a week which gave me time to moonlight. Very few of my classmates had jobs during the school year—it was just too much. What I needed was a part-time job with no regular hours that I could schedule around my research and work at on my own terms.

Painting was a lucrative undertaking—no overhead, no insurance coverage and no labor costs. I transported an extension ladder on my car and bought paint supplies at wholesale prices. I painted five houses that summer. My customers were mostly University professors. They always fed me lunch and afternoon snacks, and I listened to the top ten hit songs from a portable radio that I dragged around with me. I also dragged Lynn along when she wasn't playing with friends, so we enjoyed paint time together.

Carol's job let her take a week off for our vacation before school resumed, so we piled into the Ford and headed down to Madison on the Connecticut shore to visit Mom and Dad. On the drive, Carol glanced at me with those brown eyes full of unasked questions and unanswered doubts. About me? About us? About our future?

Hey, one year down—three to go…we're going to make it!

I resisted the urge to whistle as the hot wind from the open window whipped the collar of my shirt in a rhythm matching the beat on the radio.

"Surfin' USA",
The Beach Boys, 1963

A week with my parents, at the shore, will bring back those idyllic college days, our honeymoon, our reasons to be together on this journey. My maternal, conservative New England grandfather, Richard Hubbard Bunce for whom I was named, had built the "summer cottage" as we called it, a quaint, uninsulated three-story house with a big screened-in front porch, seven bedrooms and two and a half bathrooms. The steep-pitched, rust brown tar-shingled roof contrasted with the Cape Cod gray wood-shingled siding, occasional pieces of which would be ripped off during the late summer hurricane season. The outside showerhead that jutted from the side of the house provided the means to rinse off the sticky salt residue from the ocean and the powder-fine colored sand between the toes before entering the house. This was a cardinal rule. The house was constructed of solid maple flooring; the walls with visible vertical 3 x 3 fir supports. The focal point of the cozy living room was the heavy stone fireplace with owl andirons whose marble glass eyes glowed warm and yellow from the reflection of the fire. The living room led out to the porch through double French doors, locked at the top and bottom by sliding brass bolts, turned verdigris by the salt air. Everyone gravitated to the kitchen. Always loaded with food, Mom's kitchen welcomed family, neighbors, and guests with warmth and gracious hospitality.

In the late afternoon, as the sun drifted below the "yard-arm", the sound of Dad cracking ice cubes with his special long handled ice whacker ushered in the cocktail hour. We retired to the front porch with its unbroken view of Long Island Sound where multiple spirited conversations bristled among chomps of Vermont sharp cheddar cheese, wheat thin crackers and tiny canned mussels still dripping in oil, washed down by sips of Beefeater gin and tonic served in a tall glass clinking with ice cubes and a wedge of fresh lime for panache. The smell of little neck clams frying, lobster steaming in the pot, butter melting for the freshly shucked corn on the cob from Johnson's Farm addicted everyone who entered Mom's kitchen.

Every morning that week, Lynn, Carol and I traipsed down to the beach to build sandcastles on the sandbar at low tide, while seagulls chased hermit crabs for lunch. When I looked at Carol, I sought that exchange of glances that used to speak volumes between us, and now yielded only silence. Perhaps it was my imagination, perhaps the hectic week was too full of family to entertain intimacy, perhaps I was expecting too much from a woman who was used to my undivided attention and now settled for what I had left over from classes, studies and pressure. Perhaps she was expecting too much from a man obsessed with his professional future. Fascinated by the mechanics of surgery, focused on the possibilities of my chosen profession, and absolutely fixated on succeeding, I thought my obligation to my family required an above average performance in medical school. Or perhaps I was lying to them and to myself, as there was power in the scalpel, intimacy in the surgeon's relationship with the patient, and a guarantee of respect when you place a "Dr." before your name, and identified as a surgeon. At that time, I was running as fast as I could, in my youthful naiveté unaware that you can't outpace problems in your marriage. You need to pause enough to understand them, and then decide what to do next, if anything.

Too soon the week on the shore was over and it was back to Rochester.

"Drive carefully, son", Dad always said, as we headed back to Rochester. "You've got precious cargo there."

Lynn always stood up in the back seat and watched her grandfather wave at her as we drove away. They had a special relationship and tears flowed at every departure.

CHAPTER TEN

SECOND YEAR, AUTOPSY

*"Death sneaks up on you like the silence of
a mountain lion. Then it sinks its teeth".*
Unknown

"The End of the World"
Skeeter Davis, 1963

Second year is devoted to abnormal conditions:
pathology, parasitology, pathogenisis and pharmacology,
the language of the disease process. Taught as graduate
level science courses, the students who excelled in their
undergraduate science courses tended to do well during
these two years.

Another deceased human body began the second year,
but this time it was an autopsy. Pathology is the study of
human disease process, with termination in death.

The autopsy room was in the bowels of the hospital,
and seven of us, all second year med students, met outside
the door to garner our courage and enter as a physically
cohesive, though emotional tentative group. The hinged
metal doors swung open easily, too easily.

"Come in, gentlemen. Put on those lab coats and
stand around the table."

The prosector, Dr. Steve Fisher, a resident in pathology
and partial demi-god to a lowly second year med student,
spoke softly and in a reassuring tone. His non-descript face,

dishwater blond hair and eyebrows, pale grey eyes behind rimless glasses, belied his extraordinary influence on us. If he was aware of his importance in our lives, his demeanor did not reveal any ego. Methodical, articulate and knowledgeable, Dr. Fisher led us through the process with respect to the cadaver and to us as his associates rather than his students.

The room was cool, perhaps 60 degrees. Overhead fluorescent lights illuminated monotonous white tile floors and stark white walls. A large, rectangular metal sink with a ribbed flat area for placing freshly rinsed organs centered the room. The pathologist sliced those organs into pieces on their way to their final resting place, a glass slide with a cover slip for viewing under the microscope.

The white plastic coversheet hid the corpse, lying feet up on a slightly inclined stainless steel table. This allowed the body fluids to flow into the large drain at the end of the table. The sight of the corpse took our breath away. This body wasn't Jonas nor Judith with the painted red fingernails, but was a recently departed person; a human being, freshly dead, from causes unknown to us.

Jonas, Judith and the other cadavers had been in cold storage for weeks or even months before they became our instruments of learning. The spark of humanity was long gone before our introduction to their physical presence.

Not any more.

Suddenly, like fingernails sliding down a blackboard, the appearance of this recently deceased human being raised every hair on the back of our necks. Two days ago, anyone of us could have been that person. Alive and thinking, moving and breathing, planning and controlling, wishing and hoping for another minute, another hour and just one more day...not dead, not devoid. Medicine was driving us ever closer to that interface between life and death.

Gulp.

I hesitated to look at him, and yet couldn't avoid it.

Risking a glance around our group, I recognized similar reactions in my classmates. Blue eyes looking up at the ceiling as if the overhead popcorn insulation held the answers to unasked questions; brown eyes sliding toward the walls as if searching for a clock to check the time remaining; grey eyes, green eyes, hazel eyes looking anywhere, everywhere but the recently animated person on the table between us. But the magnetism of this human body was too powerful, and our separate glances all became focused on the matter at hand.

Dr. Fisher started the conversation as he put on his gloves, methodically arranging his instruments out of habit, and of course, exhibited no emotion whatsoever.

"This is a 58 year-old Caucasian male, a 35 pack-year smoker, the equivalent of one pack of cigarettes per day for 35 years," said Dr. Fisher as he pulled on his gloves snapping them into place.

Like a place setting at a royal dinner table, his instruments were precisely positioned on the gleaming metal Mayo stand between him and the corpse.

He continued speaking as he nonchalantly pulled the sheet down, revealing the dead body with a two-day old facial stubble, slightly open mouth revealing an absent upper right incisor tooth, and partially closed eyelids over visionless blue-gray eyes. A silent wave of emotion came over me. That could be me in 35 years, I thought to myself. Rich, Rich, you're only 23—I tried to reassure myself. You're young and healthy. Snap out of it! Once again I had to face a pre-occupation with death. Once again, I overcame it. Not always so easy. Imagine that, a sensitive guy like me wanting to become a surgeon.

"As you can see, his chest cavity is disproportionately expanded, representing long standing emphysema, from years of smoking."

Our eyes drifted down his hairy chest and scaphoid abdomen to his pubic bone, external genitalia and lower extremities and feet which angled slightly outward.

In his right hand, Dr. Fisher took the red handled dissecting blade and sliced deeply into the chest wall, a Y-shaped incision that started at either shoulder, met over the upper abdomen and descended in the mid-line to the pubis. Dark, deoxygenated blood oozed passively from the wound, which he washed away with a small, green rubber hose connected to the curved stainless steel neck of the faucet. The blood tinged water trickled over the side of the corpse's chest wall, onto the cold metal table and circled its way down into the drain. Our attention was riveted. The memories of formaldehyde stench were replaced by the unmistakable pungent odor of stale blood and cold flesh. This was the smell of death.

The incision allowed immediate entrance into the abdominal cavity, and an oscillating saw was used to briskly cut through the rib cage on both sides to facilitate entrance into the chest cavity. Attached to the overlying rib cage, a malignant tumor resisted separation, and had turned the left lung dark green and necrotic (dead tissue). With a vigorous yank of his hand, followed by a sickening crack and pop, the prosector pulled up on the rib cage segment, removing the chest wall. He placed it on the adjacent metal table.

The sounds of nervous coughing came from Bill sitting beside me. He smoked at least a pack of unfiltered Camels a day, and the sight of his future apparently caused him distinct discomfort. I looked around, and realized others in the group had the same habit as they were shaking their heads and clearing their throats, trying not to look at the devastating attack that years of cigarette smoking had caused right under their noses.

The technique used in an autopsy was an improvement over cadaver dissection, but still a far cry from my fantasy of making that very first incision on a living human being—still just a glint in my eye, but growing stronger with every passing day. From cadaver, to autopsy, to the real thing—in time Rich, in time.

The other second year courses included pharmacology (study of drug effects on pathologic conditions), bacteriology/hematology/virology, which are all inter-related in the disease process. Parasitology, the study of parasitic infestation and its rather arcane life cycle inside and outside of the human body, was perhaps the most fascinating of the courses offered that year.

The life cycles of parasites differ, species to species, but they all have common features: ingestion by a human, implantation in the gut with adult parasite formation, production of eggs which are expelled in feces, ingestion of contaminated plants by an animal, consumption of the contaminated animal by the human.

Example (taken from www.parasitology.com):   a human ingests a tapeworm larval cyst with poorly cooked, infected pork meat; the larvae escape the cysts and enter the small intestine of the human host and attach to the intestinal wall.   Small segments (proglottids) develop as the worm matures in three to four months. The adult tapeworm may live in the intestine for twenty-five years, and continually pass its eggs out with the human feces. Those eggs contaminate vegetation which is consumed by pigs. The eggs then hatch in the pig and the worm drills its way into the pig's bloodstream and ends up maturing in pig muscle.   If under-cooked pig muscle is consumed by a human, the viable eggs start the life cycle all over again.

"Honey, what are you reading?" Carol asked as she prepared dinner. I used to like studying in the kitchen in the early evening. It was a warm, friendly place and the aromas of her home cooking were a tantalizing counterpoint to the intensity of learning about the human body and its ailments. The pan of water was boiling, into which she plopped a handful of long, rigid uncooked spaghetti strands which would soon transform into a delicious plate of pasta with canned chopped clams and Kraft parmesan cheese.

"I'm studying parasites," I responded.

"You mean those yucky creatures that feed off of your intestines?" Carol asked, then paused. "Tell me about them, Rich."

"Well, the ugliest of the bunch are called roundworms, especially ascaris."

"What's the Latin name?" Carol's intellect carried far beyond the norm. "It helps me visualize it better."

"It's called Ascaris lumbricoides, and lays up to 200,000 eggs a day. The eggs will pass out in the excrement of an infected animal, say a fox or a raccoon. If a human then eats a fruit or vegetable contaminated by the excrement, the eggs will end up in his small intestine where they molt into larvae."

"Then what?" Carol prodded with increasing interest.

"How's the spaghetti coming?" I asked with increasing interest.

"Fine, fine. Tell me more", she implored.

"Okay. Well, the larvae then drill their way through the wall of the intestine and into the bloodstream where they are carried to the lungs. Now comes the gross part. They so irritate the lining of the lungs that the person starts to cough them up. But he swallows some, too, and once the larvae make it back into the intestine for the second time, trouble starts big time."

"Like what?" she asked.

"Don't overcook the spaghetti." I was getting hungry.

"Oh, stop it! Continue," she demanded.

"The larvae then morph into an adult which attaches to the inside lining (mucosa) of the intestine and start sucking nutrients and blood to grow and thrive. And to pass eggs by the millions out that person's rear end."

"Oh, that's totally disgusting!" She returned her attention to the boiling water on the stove. "Tell me more."

"OK. The professor presented a case today where a female patient looked in the toilet bowl after going to the bathroom and saw three worms wriggling around in the water."

Carol moved to the sink and dumped the spaghetti into a colander to drain. "And then what?"

"The worms were over a foot long."

Carol grabbed some tongs and began lifting spaghetti from the colander to drop on the plate she held in her other hand. "And?"

"Well, the patient screamed. Her husband rushed into the bathroom and saw his wife jumping up and down, pointing at the toilet. He plucked one of the wriggling bastards out of the toilet and dropped it into a jar." I noticed Carol wasn't looking so good...her mouth was making odd motions and she appeared to be swallowing a lot. "It, the tapeworm, was still wriggling....?"

"Yeah," I responded. "Kind of like the spaghetti you were stirring in the pot!"

Carol shoved the plate full of pasta at me before putting her hand up to her mouth and dashing past me into the bathroom.

I heard her retching, and decided not to discuss parasitology anymore, ever.

Tested throughout the year, at the end of my second year, I added up the number of hours I had spent taking exams from college through second year med school—over 680 hours of solid exam taking! Come on, summer!

The second summer was similar to the first.

I painted up a storm, and my lab research went well.

Interested in the phenomenon of shock, a state in which blood flow is so reduced that it can no longer supply vital organs with needed substances such as oxygen and glucose, without which these organs cease to function and shock becomes irreversible, resulting in death; I spent my research time trying to determine what compensatory mechanisms the body recruits in order to survive, and what fails when it doesn't.

There are many different causes of shock such as loss of blood by hemorrhage (hemorrhagic shock), or damage to the heart from a heart attack (cardiac shock), or overwhelming bacterial infection (septic shock). Despite the different causes, the effects of all these different types of shock at the cellular level appear to be very similar, and it was the possibility of a set of common factors that I was investigating. If this were the case, the basic principles in treating all kinds of shock would be the same. This was not an original concept by any means, but it allowed me a chance to become deeply involved in a challenging problem from both the experimental and theoretical aspects.

The experience I gained in the rat lab was learning the scientific approach to a specified problem, in preparation for eventually publishing an article in some medical journal. The process one takes is detailed, compulsive and methodical. In short, the order of investigation starts with a theory, proposal or assumption, followed by the method of approach, leading to a set of results which finally must be reconciled with the original theory. Sounds boring, but conclusions can be explosive. However, my preferences were definitely pointing in the direction of clinical surgery and patient care, not research or academia. Lab did not excite me. The high drama of human interaction on a surgical level did.

The last two years of med school are the clinical years. Under the supervision of interns, residents, and faculty, students are assigned to individual patients. They learn on the job by assisting in and observing the diagnosis and treatment of these patients. Additional learning takes place in formal lectures and teaching rounds, during which students discuss their patients as well as those of other students on their particular service (e.g. pediatrics, psychiatry).

The clinical years immerse the students more and more into a less structured, less mathematically exact environment where observation, assimilation and judgment come into play. To excel in these last two years requires learning how to arrive at correct conclusions, often based on subtle and incomplete information. The crux of superior medical education is not only to equip students with the knowledge they will need to care for patients, but also with the ability to form sound judgments.

CHAPTER ELEVEN

THIRD YEAR:
BEYOND THE BODY

"You can't let praise or criticism get to you.
It's a weakness to get caught up in either one."
John Wooden, *college basketball coach*

"Come Go with Me",
Del-Vikings, 1957

Now, finally, began the glorious third year of med school. No more cadavers, no more autopsies, no more grilling exams (for a while anyhow). Two years of rote memory gave way to a higher level of observation and behavioral integration. Even though this was medicine as practiced in the 1960's when the word "holistic" was not yet part of the vernacular, the emphasis was not solely on body parts. We were trained to observe in minute detail the physical elements of our patients, to note the normal and to focus on the variations from normal in order to create a diagnosis. Beyond that was the context of the patient's, "life style", another phrase popularized in the late twentieth century, which could lend clues when their body refused to give up any.

For the third year medical student, armed with two years of data, spring loaded to fire on his first target, the excitement in finally having access to a living, breathing whole specimen to study was hard to contain. Outside the hospital, we glanced at the red-faced overweight individual in line at the post office and shook our heads in dismay at the probable pending myocardial infarction, like 7:59 AM on an alarm clock set for 8:00 AM. The little old lady with the cane in her right hand and decidedly left arm and leg weakness undoubtedly had suffered a right brain thrombotic occlusion (stroke) of a tiny cerebral artery. The chain-smoking dinner guest's rough voice raised the specter of laryngeal carcinoma. Sitting next to him was his wife and the sound of the ice cubes rattling in her water glass betrayed a diagnosis of Parkinson's disease. To the trained eye, every day events will reveal pathology that leaps out like a single oak tree in a forest full of firs.

A flash forward: inside your body

Certain habits go hand in hand, like a young couple walking down the street in love. Not always, but often enough to make the surgeon aware. Smoking and drinking love each other, simpatico, buddies to the end. Furthermore, almost without exception, patients will minimize their habits. Like a good attorney who knows the answer to every question he asks, I prefer the indirect approach. In my pre-op evaluation, I need maximum information about the patient, so I run down the list we call "review of systems".

"Mrs. Jones (hypothetical), do you smoke?" Mrs. Jones has already given me the answer: I can smell smoke in her hair as I listen to her heart; I hear expiratory wheezes in her lungs when I listen to her chest; her voice is a bit raspy and lower in tone than expected for her age; her skin shows premature sagging and has diminished turgor (elasticity) on gentle pinch; her chest wall shows abnormal expansion in the anterior-posterior dimension (front to back), the result of damaged lung tissue struggling desperately to increase volume in order to compensate for decrease in functional ability; her resting pulse rate is higher than normal, the result of a heart trying to pump more blood through those damn lungs to exchange oxygen and carbon dioxide in the right amounts; an ever so subtle change in her nail beds called clubbing, a sentinel of insidious pulmonary disease, and in her lips and gums that betray a trace of purplish discoloration due to lower O_2 content in tiny arteries (arterioles); and in her body habitus (constitution) which often betrays a decreased appetite for food in place of an increased appetite for cigarettes.

"Well, Dr. German, I do smoke, but I'm down to half a pack a day." Translation: Mrs. Jones has been smoking one and a half packs a day for 25 years (known as 37 pack years) and is struggling to stay at a pack a day.

"And Mrs. Jones, do you get short of breath going up stairs?"

"Sometimes I do, yes."

And there it is, staring me in the face—I have placed her pre-op chest x-ray on my view box, and the inspiratory film shows marked lung volume expansion, flattened diaphragms bilaterally, and hyperaeration of the darkened lung fields. Translation: moderate emphysema and an increased anesthetic risk because of it. That will not make Dr. Anesthesiologist very happy.

"And Mrs. Jones, do you drink?"

Again, I suspect the answer. She has prominent facial telangectases (prominent, red vascularity) on her nose and cheeks. I quickly peruse her lab report in front of me.

Her pro time (clotting ability) is upper limits of normal, perhaps a telltale sign of compromised liver function due to early alcoholic cirrhosis.

"I drink occasionally, Dr. German. Perhaps 3 or 4 drinks a week." I suspect more.

Fast forward to the day of her surgery, a gall bladder removal (cholecystectomy). Mrs. Jones is on the OR table, anesthetized and asleep, prepped and draped. The surgeon makes the incision. Blood rushes up the side of the cold steel, Bard-Parker knife blade, but lacks the bright coloration I expect — emphysema rears its ugly head. The abnormally thin layer of fat lacks the usual bright yellow appearance of healthy adipose tissue, and the skin exhibits poor turgor (poor elasticity) due to years of smoking which has relentlessly broken down the collagen and elastin in the dermis. To be absolutely blunt, we call this "PPP", or piss poor protoplasm which presages a potentially difficult post-operative healing process. The knife drives deeper through the fascia and break into the abdominal cavity.

"Well, well gentlemen, look what we have here,." I say to myself. The liver, normally smooth and a deep reddish-brown, is pale, contracted and hobnailed. It has a bumpy cobblestoned appearance on the surface which is studded by 1 cm in size, lumpy islands of non-functional scar tissue. Translation: alcoholic cirrhosis not due to "3 or 4 drinks a week", but probably 5 times that.

Our dear Mrs. Jones is walking down a predetermined path, hand and hand with her 2 best friends, cigarettes and alcohol. Slow suicide is staring her in the face.

*"The eye sees only what the mind is
prepared to comprehend."*
Robertson Davies, author

Anecdote from John Stuart Mill (1806-1873):
*A young boy and his father. A street in London, 1813.
Window shops. A fertile testing ground for a precocious mind.
The boy glanced at the window displays, not with passing interest or idle curiosity. Nor even with childish excitement. Rather,
with a voracious though disciplined determination to commit everything he saw to memory. And not just the objects, but detailed
characteristics of the objects themselves—color, size, shape, texture,
pattern—as well their relationship to each other. He looked away
and recited what he had seen to his father, until he became so pro-
ficient at this game that a quick glance yielded a lengthy and
accurate verbal reproduction. The objects, of course, were an academic vehicle. From objects to thoughts, from thoughts to ideas and
the transition was made smoothly, simultaneously, imperceptibly.
His was the unique talent to grasp the most subtle of facts, to per-
ceive their intricacies and provide their associations.*

Astute observation had not yet become a discipline
with me; not unlike many in my generation, the intensity
of my observation related to my degree of interest. At the
end of the pre-clinical years, this became rudely apparent
after a brief interview with a patient.

After taking a deep breath, straightening my tie and
my spine, I confidently opened the door to the patient's
room and stepped inside. My untrained attention like a
diamond cutter's eyepiece focused on the body in the
washed out hospital gown lying prone on the bed in front

of me. But all I saw was a thatch of badly dyed red hair behind the covers of the latest best seller she was apparently reading. Would she ask me a question? And if so, how would I answer, what could I say? I'm not a doctor, only one in training. I can't ask her to wait a couple of years for my answer. Did she know I was a fraud in a starched white coat, whose only caduceus was engraved on my jacket not on a sheepskin...not yet.

After a weak smile and a mumbled greeting, I snapped my fingers as if I had forgotten something important, turned on my heel and escaped back into the hallway....right into the attending physician who was on his way in to observe my performance.

"That was fast," his baritone voice tinged with more than a hint of sarcasm. Whippet thin, a face like the business end of a razor, his Italian heritage was revealed in his long, aquiline nose, olive skin and thick, dark hair in stark contrast to his colorless surroundings. "*Mis*ter German," (was it my imagination or did he draw out the "Miss" in Mister?), he said. "Please reconstruct everything you saw and heard in the hospital room which would contribute to an accurate evaluation of this patient's status."

I began to stammer, desperately thinking of an explanation for my hasty retreat, finally resorting to the truth, I responded. "Uh, I haven't evaluated her status yet...I, uh, wanted to return to the hall to gather my thoughts before interacting with a patient."

"Not a bad idea," he said with a smile.

I stood there smiling stupidly at him, until he shoved open the door and stepped inside, holding it open for me to follow him.

This attending physician gifted me with a fine example in patient evaluation that day. Not just the clinical diagnosis, but more important, all the subtle clues which so vividly reveal the nature of the patient. At first, my untrained attention was diluted by strong subjective involvement. The details of the room itself went unnoticed, partly because of my obvious fixation on the patient, and partly because I never considered the significance of a patient's immediate setting—namely that one is reflected in his or her surroundings. A person leaves the fingerprints of his personality on the environment in a multiplicity of ways. The absence of an action or an object may be of greater significance than the presence of another.

So it was to these matters of detail that I had to apply myself. For instance, this patient's room was well lighted and the shades up; there was no special duty nurse, IV bottles or catheters; and she was propped up in bed reading a book—all indications that her medical problem was stable. There were four or five get-well cards sitting on the bedside table, surrounding a pretty flower arrangement. This implied support from family or close friends and a home to return to. The latter assumption was supported by a wedding ring and a letter lying on her bed with a local postmark and return address bearing the same last name as the patient. No rosary beads or religious cross present so she was probably not Catholic. She was reading In Cold Blood by Truman Capote, wore appropriate make-up and an attractive hairstyle—probably above average intelligence. A cornflower blue robe and matching slippers lay near the bed indicating an ambulatory status. No crutches or cane were present.

Beside the clipboard which showed an afebrile (absence of any fever) course hung a sign reading "bland diet" and a bottle of Maalox with a whitened spoon resting on the table. Diagnosis—peptic ulcer. That would fit. She was slightly overweight, about 42, probably married to a well-to-do man (she was in a private room) and probably had high school aged children. All of this was subject for observation in the few seconds before doctor and patient greeted each other, in the brief time walking from the door to the bedside.

Information had been gathered, assumptions made and further information sought so as to support or alter those assumptions—a continuing application of the scientific approach: facts, hypothesis and experimentation.

Experimentation occurs in all forms of doctor-patient interaction, i.e., the interview, the physical exam and testing. In this patient's case, the interview supplemented information and supported or refuted hypothesis. It was not only important to learn about this woman's physical ailment but also about her whole being: how she thought, what analogies she made, what selective and seemingly unrelated bits of personal information she offered from what appeared to be the absolute periphery of the problem.

A wise doctor once told me that the time you start to diagnose a patient is when you first see him getting out of his car across the street from your office, or standing next to you in the elevator, or when you hear him speak to your secretary—in other words, from the first moment you observe the patient in any way he presents himself. So it was to this encompassing approach that I had to apply myself. The key is accurate observation coupled with logical reasoning. A person can make a wrong conclusion from the correct facts, but he can never make a correct conclusion from the wrong facts; or no facts at all.

One day in psychiatry class this process became evident. With her consent, a middle-aged woman was placed alone in a small room for observation. We sat on the other side of a one-way mirror in a separate room observing her. There was a blackboard with some colored chalk, a few magazines, some books, and an ash tray in the room. She sat quietly reading a magazine and smoked a cigarette and coughed once.

After 20 minutes she left. The professor asked us to write down every fact about her we could remember—wedding ring, no make-up, neat hairstyle, an unnatural shade of blonde hair, smoked with her left hand, had a pleasant expression, breathed regularly and quietly, looked at one weekly magazine. From these observations we were asked to give our impressions of her personal life. Married, right handed, high school education, above average intelligence, dyed hair, average income, children, inactive socially, non-athletic, one car family. A surprising number of these assumptions were correct. As I remember we were wrong about her education as she was pursuing her Bachelors Degree here at the University and had no children. Perhaps she would have selected a parenting magazine to read had she had children, or a tennis or golf magazine if she played either sport. Every behavioral act is selective, no matter how mundane. A word, an act, a joke, an analogy—always selected in favor of other choices, though not necessarily on a conscious level. This premise of selectivity allows rather accurate predictions of a person's behavior.

During my third year I had an interesting case where observation played a key role. A thin, rather disheveled graying middle-aged woman came into med school clinic and nervously asked to talk to me in private. I invited her into the office and as she sat down, she turned to watch me close the door. Several seconds passed without me saying anything, allowing her the opportunity to initiate the conversation.

She said nothing.

When I asked why she had come in for a consultation she said, "I can't tell you."

At first I thought she was simply reflecting her own emotional confusion, though most people will respond with "I don't know". In fact, she was implying the diagnosis in that first sentence, though I was not perceptive enough to realize it at that moment.

Her reluctance to speak forced me to ask more direct questions, probing into her personal life.

"Who do you live with at home?"

"Do you get along with your children?"

"Who or what bothers you the most?" and so on.

She responded in single syllables, and then refused to continue. I missed the significance of that as well.

I felt my discomfort rising and my patience falling as the strained, unproductive and one-sided interview continued for 20 long minutes. A water pipe in the wall began hissing steam in the middle of my next question.

"What's that noise?" She interrupted me. Shrinking into herself, an expression of extreme anxiety and suspicion on her face, she whipped her head back and forth searching for the source of the noise. "Someone's listening?"

She was unable to distinguish reality from non-reality and her inappropriate suspicion reflected a psychotic fear of her environment. The pipe was simply a coincidental event. Eventually, she would have chosen something else if not the hissing pipe. And in fact she had done that when she first entered the office and turned to make sure that I closed the door. She was a paranoid schizophrenic. Consistent with her paranoia was the fear that certain people were after her, trying to harm her. The dilemma she faced was the intensity of her paranoia, since she feared these people were listening to our conversation and therefore to her accusations. This is why she had said "I can't tell you."

Perhaps more than any other subject in the medical curriculum, psychiatry pointed out the complexities of human relationships not only with others, but with themselves. Until this course our instruction had focused on the structure, systems, and normal and abnormal of the human body. Psychiatry goes beyond the physiology of the brain into the behavior produced by that organ. This course gave us an appreciation for the need of a broader approach to a patient. In those days, the medical school at Rochester was known for this approach to the practice of medicine.

The integration of behavior within a global pathophysiologic environment ("internal milieu") was the hallmark of a Rochester education. By whatever name, today this is an accepted approach to health and wellness. Because of my exposure to psychiatry at Rochester, I became aware of that perspective earlier than many of my colleagues. It had been instructive, and if nothing else, it had humbled me.

As a med student, you remember certain pearls that were passed down from the "Gods of Wisdom", your professors. One such pearl referred to the exact moment you begin to diagnose a patient. Another that has stuck with me all these years is that a doctor must not be offended by disproportionate criticism nor become arrogant with unjustified praise.

One conspicuous example was the first case of litigation that I became aware of in my medical career. The general surgeon on call, a professor of mine, was on his way home to the Rochester suburbs when he was called back to the emergency room. The patient was a 42 year-old female chronic alcoholic who had developed liver cirrhosis. Consequently, tributary channels had developed to divert blood away from the scarred liver. These channels had become dangerously swollen along the walls of the esophagus and suddenly burst one night on an alcoholic binge. She was rushed to the hospital vomiting up mouthfuls of bright red blood and large clots. She was bleeding into her stomach and was in shock. Blood was sent to the lab for type and cross and IV's were established in both arms. A large rubber tube well lubricated with KY jelly was placed in her nose and gently eased down her esophagus and into her stomach. Through this tube blood was evacuated and ice water instilled in attempt to constrict the bleeding vessels, X-rays were taken, a Foley catheter placed in her bladder and the OR alerted. After multiple transfusions, she finally stopped bleeding. This in itself was a minor triumph. She was stabilized and then taken to surgery. The operation is always dangerous especially in someone in her poor state of health. If she had no surgery, chances were high that she would succumb to another fatal hemorrhage.

The operation was performed with her full consent and knowledge of the risk involved. During the case as in any major operation, small straps with metal plates were attached to her wrists and ankles in order to monitor her EKG. The operation, though long and tedious, was successful. She had passed two major crises, which claimed the lives of many similar patients, and now had a second chance at life absent any further drinking.

The only complication was that one of the rubber straps had been on too tight, causing a small area of skin irritation on her wrist which fully healed within one week. For this "personal injury" she sued the hospital for $50,000. Of course, the case was dismissed but I will never forget the incredulous expression on the face of the surgeon when he learned of the lawsuit. Such is medicine and such is the ability to maintain a stoic demeanor and carry on.

Third year med students wore slacks, shirt and tie, and donned crisp white jackets with a stethoscope tucked in the left pocket which made us look, and feel, like real life doctors. Eli Lilly, the pharmaceutical company, had given each of us, all 72 students, a black leather medical bag containing our own Littman stethoscope, tuning fork, reflex hammer and oto(ear)/opthalmascope—not a cheap gift, and an amazement to me. The subliminal message was, "Don't forget us when you start writing prescriptions in two years".

As soon as we could choose our electives, I made a bee-line to surgery and the OR with all the enthusiasm of a high school student at the Junior Prom. The first operation that I observed was a tonsillectomy—the room was dark, all overhead lights were off and the surgeon had a headlight that was shining directly into the open mouth of an anesthetized 10 year-old girl. Everything was in whispers, the surgeon putting out his hand and the scrub nurse gently handing him the appropriate instrument. Like clockwork, in and out of the mouth, first one instrument, then another, all in preparation for amputating the base of the tonsil with a snare.

Out of the corner of my eye I saw the float nurse sitting on a stool reading a magazine and looking complacent and bored. Christ! This was the most exciting thing I had ever seen—was she crazy? She was missing the whole thing! In reality, what I was missing was that she had seen this a hundred times over. It was my first OR tingle and it only got better as third year flew by and I racked up one operation after another as an observer. My cup runneth over!

Dr. Jim Adamson was a piece of work. An associate professor of surgery, and I believe of Armenian descent, his thick black hair shoved his straight across hairline to within kissing distance of his football-like black eyebrows which hung suspended over deep set, riveting dark brown eyes. Short tempered, quick witted, flamboyant and direct, his teaching style was to allow a med student little more than a nano second response to an anatomic question, and then out of impatience provide his own answer in machine gun fire rapidity. Just as light follows a straight line as the shortest path between two points, Adamson would provide an unbroken, verbal barrage as the shortest distance between question and answer.

After one in our group gave a confused response to a question during his allotted nano second, Adamson burst out, "Dave, you know ice cream vendors wear white, too. You might consider that instead of medicine!" Dave melted into his seat like an ice cream cone; the rest of us froze.

For some strange reason I got along pretty well with Adamson. I never felt the sting of a demeaning comment, and his impatience came across as a prudent teaching method that I seemed to resonate with rather easily. In fact, I took it as a compliment that perhaps he felt I could keep up with him and achieve. A year later, when I was applying for a surgical internship, a fellow med student told me he overheard Adamson say, "German will be a good surgeon. We want him in the program." Not surprisingly, I was accepted to the surgical internship program a few months later.

Indeed, Adamson invited me to assist on a hernia operation (herniorrhaphy). Or so I thought.

He ran down every excruciating detail of the operation, from the direction and depth of the inguinal (groin) incision to the repair and final closure, an 11 minute dissertation which I tried to digest as best possible. As we walked into the OR, scrubbed and gowned, he directed me to the surgeon's side of the table, while he moved opposite me on the assistant side. Jesus! He's letting me do the case!

"Knife," I hesitantly gestured to the scrub nurse.

"Now remember what I told you," Adamson directed.

With some trepidation, I took the Bard-Parker in my right hand, adjusted it appropriately, and made a perfect incision.

Or so I thought.

One nano second later, before the first molecule of hemoglobin had a chance to stain the side of my blade, Adamson shouted, "Stop! Stop! You just did exactly what I told you NOT to do!!" It seems I had made the incision one millimeter off center. I suffered through the case in a somewhat bumbling manner, until, out of sheer frustration at my ponderous, pachyderm-like progress, he grabbed the suture and rapidly completed the repair. He directed the scrub nurse to count down in 30 second increments, since he considered it a personal insult to take longer than 28 minutes on a herniorraphy. "It will ruin my reputation," Adamson fumed.

With furious speed, needle holder flying, knots tied and squared, I had a hard time just keeping up cutting the sutures while Adamson did everything else. As the nurse counted down, "10-9-8-7...", he flung his arms up in the air to signal completion of the case in just under 28 minutes, much like a rodeo cowboy hog-tying a steer.

> *"Personality has the power to open many doors, but character must keep them open".*
>
> Unknown

Regardless of the area of practice, the medical practitioner's written record might as well be stone tablets. The doctor is in charge of the patient throughout the treatment process. He or she captains their ship, and is ultimately responsible for whatever occurs on his watch. If the patient is referred to a specialist, then that doctor assumes total responsibility for the treatment.

When the internist makes the diagnosis, the referral will determine the course of treatment. If you go to an oncologist, you will receive chemo; if you go to a radiologist, you will receive radiation; and if you go to a surgeon—-expect surgery.

Academic, experience, and intelligence defines which protocol applies to which treatment. The internist will identify the facts, the results of the tests in each situation, and prescribe the appropriate treatment. When there is a grey zone in a diagnosis, the internist is entitled to an opinion and will back it up with studies, results and recommendation.

The doctor's responsibility is to provide the best advice available as to treatment. When the patient moves from a general practitioner into a specialist's hands, and from there to a sub-specialist, increased scrutiny on the prescribed treatment accompanies the patient.

In 1970, the "cowboy" was more acceptable, because there was less scrutiny and follow up unless something went wrong, very wrong. In those days, medical personnel were left to police themselves. Now, the increased involvement of insurance companies and government intervention into the practice of medicine creates a "fishbowl" atmosphere for every health practitioner. Over the years, "Big Brother" has slowly insinuated itself into the practice of medicine. BMQA, or the Bureau of Medical Quality Assurance, was a euphemism for a government agency we called "the Gestapo"—screw up and face a very unpleasant experience of scrutiny and discipline.

First, there are too many reliable pre-tests to determine the ailment and the appropriate treatment for a doctor to abuse the system to make his car payment. Secondly, doctors are people with all of the motivators found in every profession: competition, jealousy, ambition. These less than honorable motivations tend to keep everyone honest. If there is a pattern of not following the accepted protocol, criticism is sure to pinpoint this aberrant behavior. Finally, there are committees in every community to hold a health practitioner's feet to the fire if/when there is cause for concern.

Unless they were born with a scalpel for a hand, or with X-ray vision, or an obsession with inanimate objects, most undergraduate doctors have only a vague idea of what they specialize in after graduation. Since we rotated through all of the specialties, the final decision was made over a gradual period of time. However, whether your grandfather received chickens for the successful delivery of a baby in a rural community, or your mother's aspirations for "My son, the doctor" on Park Avenue combating the aging process with a Dermatology practice, or your dreams of probing the motivations of aberrant behavior of serial killers, your personality contributes to your choice of practice.

Your selection of a specialty may depend upon the relationship you want with your patients; whether you want to work **with** them or **on** them. Those of us who require immediate gratification and relish high risk, short term goals are drawn to the high intensity specialties, surgery being the most obvious choice. Add a good pair of hands, compassion and a dash of compulsion and you have the makings of a surgeon.

Within each specialty there is an element of risk, some more visible than others and the narrower the specialty—- the more intense your focus.

Those doctors who gravitate to intensity of experience will be drawn toward those specialties where immediate life and death decisions must be made...which is why many surgeons have pilots' licenses.

The more contemplative, deliberate doctors prefer a professional life as an internist, psychiatrist or oncologist where patience is definitely a virtue. In other words, the usual lack of dire urgency that surgeons thrive on allows the non-surgeon practitioner the luxury of patience.

Pediatric oncology requires a very special gift. A gentle, caring personality, tremendous courage and empathetic people skills are necessary to work to affect a cure, cheer a remission, or console parents after a child's passing. The gift of this practice are the occasional miracles—-and yes, they do happen—-and it takes a very special person to go to work day after day in the expectation of another one.

Quietly, and behind closed doors, that physician has to reach deep down and somehow deal with the most powerful loss a physician has to face—the death of a child entrusted to his or her care.

I have had the privilege of training under many of the finest clinical professors in medicine. All possessed penetrating intellect. Some transcended intellect and radiated lasting principles of life. And a handful, a very few indeed, rose above all the rest. They instilled an aura of excellence and professionalism that went far beyond the tangible, and left one inspired for a life-long attempt to emulate.

Dr. James Phelps, a pediatric oncologist, was such a man. Tall, dark hair, youthful face and trim stature, he spoke in gentle tones and never raised his voice. He came up with revolutionary ideas for treating children with cancer, and had a reassuring demeanor that put his young patient and their parents at ease. He had the ability to soothe child and parent alike, and gave them confidence in his superior ability to provide a cure, prolong the quality of life or ease the inevitable transition without fear. The lasting effect this compassionate physician, teacher and mentor left upon me was awareness of the patient. Would that this caring man could have eased my best friend Binky through his own inevitable transition so many years ago.

Specialties...disciplines...personalities.

The ego-driven surgeon's dictum is "A chance to cut is a chance to cure". This says something of a surgeon's personality. A physician in internal medicine or psychiatry, for instance, must be less anxious for immediate results, and receives gratification from extended, longer term involvement. There are "slang" medical terms that describe various specialties and often give subtle insight as to the type of gratification one receives in his field—pedipods (pediatricians), plastic men (cosmetic and reconstructive plastic surgeons), zappers (radiation therapy), tinker toys (paraphernalia used by orthopedic surgeons to erect metal frames, weights and supports for broken limbs), plumbers (urologists), "butts-R-us" (proctologists), and so on.

The disciplines of pathology, radiology and anesthesiology traditionally demanded far less continuous patient interaction, and for whatever reasons, certain personalities gravitate to these fields. Anesthesiology does indeed bring physician and patient into a close relationship, one in which the patient entrusts his life, as in every other interaction a person has with health practitioners. The interactive part of the relationship with the anesthesiologist is a very brief duration, usually conducted in the pre-op holding station and lasting only a few minutes. The patient is anxious, fearful, and not their normal selves, the anesthesiologist is observant, professional and reassuring. After surgery, the anesthesiologist insures stability of the patient in the recovery room, again a relationship lasting only a few minutes...when the patient is in various stages of consciousness. In between those two brief interludes, the anesthesiologist renders the patient unconscious with the wonders of modern anesthetics.

Until recently, radiology involved very little patient-physician interaction. "Old school" radiology meant reading x-rays, reporting the findings, and then going home to dinner. This is not to dismiss the importance of the ability to read an x-ray, rather to illustrate the increased involvement in treatment options of the modern radiologist. With the advance of interventional radiology, the radiologist performs multiple invasive procedures: insertion of long needles under CT scan guidance to biopsy an organ; to drain body fluids such as a collection of blood, bile or cystic fluid; insertion of catheters into the vascular system with injection of dye for arteriographic or venographic evaluation; establishing venous access for the purpose of providing high potency calories (total parenteral nutrition, or TPN) into the major vein of the body—— the superior vena cava.

Treatment depends on the reliability of the x-rays, and it is incumbent upon the radiologist to scrutinize the quality of those x-rays. If they are not acceptable, the radiologist will insist on re-takes until the results are deemed adequate for an accurate interpretation. He cannot be legally excused from missing a diagnosis based on an inferior x-ray taken under his authority. Still, the patient-radiologist interaction remains very limited. In fact, in most cases the two never meet. The radiologist, a talented technician, aids the attending physician who is primarily responsible for the patient.

The most limited exposure to patients belongs to the pathologist. Most of the pathologist's time is spent in the lab examining tissue under the microscope, tissue that was sent from a doctor's office as a biopsy, or from surgery as a re-sected organ. On occasion, the pathologist performs a bone marrow biopsy on an in-patient, but the verbal exchange is obviously very brief, if it occurs at all (the patient may be somnolent or comatose).

The pathologist looks at parts of a patient, rarely the entire person.

The obvious exception is the autopsy, definitely a non-verbal experience.

This is not to say that such physicians purposely gravitate to these three fields that afford minimal doctor-patient interaction. In fact, these physicians tend to be very personable and balanced. Rather, they choose to gravitate to a specialty that appeals to them and is personally rewarding.

Popular literature and entertainment in general portrays the surgeon as a temperamental, yet talented, loner. The cowboy of medicine who rides into town with a gun belt full of silver bullets, challenges the cancer, the injury, the diseased organ to a showdown. On Main Street at high noon, the towns' folk watch from a safe distance. They admire the hero's skill as he vanquishes the enemy with a quick draw and a few well aimed shots. Then he blows on his six guns, returns them to his holster, turns on his heel, remounts his horse, and rides out of town…into the sunset.

Most of us don't feel that way.

But all of us feel.

Impressions to the contrary, some of the most impersonal, apparently detached physicians I know are surgeons. Perhaps they require distance from the emotional demands of sick patients and worried families in order to perform the necessary surgery. Perhaps they are socially awkward under any circumstances. Perhaps the intensity required to hold a throbbing organ in their hands, or re-attach a limb successfully, or restore sight to an artist's eye, or hearing to a composer's ear, or return sensation to a carpenter's hands, or the smile to a mother's lips cannot accommodate a charming personality, or a comforting bedside manner familiar to media surgeons.

I know why surgery was my choice, my only choice. I wanted to be a mechanic of the human body, a great mechanic, with the ability to make the right diagnosis, intervene physically, face the challenge and correct the problem expeditiously. It seemed so eminently satisfying to me, from start to finish.

"Baby, I'm Yours",
Barbara Lewis, 1965

The most physically intimate relationship you can have with another human being, surgery is a one way interaction. The scalpel penetrates the patient's skin, allowing access to the internal organs. Once inside the abdominal cavity, the surgeon's knowledge of the patient's body guides him to a cure and his hands remedy the problem. Sutures reseal the interior, and the healing begins.

Once the patient's internal organs are exposed, they may inform the surgeon of wellness or disease, function or malfunction, life or death. The surgeon carries away more detailed information about his patient and his future than the patient will ever know about himself.

It is a mixed blessing.

CHAPTER TWELVE

REALITY CHECK

"In matters of style, swim with the current.
In matters of principle, stand like a rock."
Thomas Jefferson, 3rd U.S. President

"Do You Believe In Magic?,
Lovin' Spoonful, 1965

The weeks turned into months as the year flew by. I was used to diagnosing pathology in my patients, not in my own family. That was about to change. Following my routine, I fit in an hour to shoot some hoops with Bill and Frank before going home to a warm supper and the two women in my life.

After a quick shower and a short bike ride on slick streets, I arrived home feeling really, really good about life, the future, and my family's place in it. I took the steps three at a time to our apartment, and smelled the aroma of my favorite meal drifting into the hallway...it turned out that aroma came from the apartment next door to ours.

Putting my medical bag down as soon as I walked in the door, slipping off my slicker, and then my lab coat, and carefully hanging both of them up in the hall closet, I called out to Carol. "Hi, honey—"

"Rich, hush..." She turned with her index finger to her lips and nodded toward Lynn who was asleep on the couch. "She has a fever…so I let her curl up there until you came home to kiss her good night."

I approached my daughter as quietly as possible on a wooden floor that squeaked with each footstep. Apparently she didn't hear me, as she didn't wake up when I leaned over and pressed my lips to her forehead. Hot. Yes, that's a fever all right.

Standing up, I walked back to Carol and answered her unasked question, "She'll be all right—-probably just a cold, or the spring flu." I announced in my best diagnostic voice. She smiled, apparently reassured, and then returned her attention to the Chef Boyardee canned spaghetti she was heating on the gas stove in front of her.

After dinner, I was studying and Carol was reading when a quivering voice from my 3 year-old jarred me from the depths of the porta-hepatus.

"Daddy, I don't feel so good."

"What honey, what's wrong?" I picked Lynn up and sat her in my lap.

"Carol, she feels warm." I felt a flutter of concern as I felt her forehead with my hand. "Where's the thermometer?"

"Daddy, my throat hurts and I feel sick." Her head flopped against my shoulder and she partially closed her eyes.

"Honey, can you look at Daddy?"

"No, my neck hurts," as she pressed her head into my shoulder.

Oh boy! My mind silently raced through the differential diagnoses, a list of middle ear infection, adenitis, tonsillitis, upper respiratory infection, pharyngitis, chicken pox, all possible causes for Lynn's symptoms in descending order of probability. I kept readjusting the diagnostic possibilities as I carefully examined her hot, limp body; throat slightly red, mild cervical lymphadenopathy (neck lymph node swelling), chest clear, heart tachycardic (rapid rate), diminished cervical range of motion (neck stiffness). And I kept coming back to that same possibility—meningitis.

"Honey, Mommy and I are taking you to the hospital so a doctor can check you out."

"But you're a doctor, Daddy".

"Well, almost, honey, but I'm not a kid doctor and I want a kid doctor to look at you to make sure your throat is okay."

"Okay, Daddy," and she fell asleep in my arms as we made the quick drive to the hospital.

"Carol, grab my jacket..." I said, referring to the windbreaker over the back of a chair near the front door.

Instead, she grabbed my white coat and jammed my stethoscope into the pocket. Puzzled for a moment, I understood what she was doing as soon as she looked at me. Her brows lifted over dark brown eyes, her mouth tight in grim determination, her hands shaky with fear she helped me into my lab coat around our sleeping daughter.

Carol drove the short distance to the hospital, as I held my feverish child in my arms. Pulling up at the ER entrance, I struggled out of the car with my precious cargo while Carol parked the car in the space reserved for the ER patients.

As soon as I identified myself and my daughter, a nurse ushered us right into a curtained examination room. A few minutes later, Carol joined us. I gently lowered Lynn to the middle of the hospital bed, but when I tried to release her she whimpered and held on tighter, so I picked her up again to wait the arrival of the doctor.

"Rich? What is it?" Carol asked in a voice indicating she didn't really want an answer.

I was about to list the possibilities when a nurse with a horizontal blue stripe on her nurse's cap pulled open the curtain surrounding us. The pediatric resident, "John Byrd, M.D." according to the nametag clipped to his lab coat pocket, entered with a gentle smile and introduced himself with a softly reassuring voice.

His brown hair in a short crew cut, blue eyes made bluer by his button down collared blue shirt, and Republican Red tie; he filled out his bright white lab coat with the confidence of an athlete. His short compact stature indicated a running back on his undergraduate team, or maybe a Varsity rugby scrum hooker. The nurse entered to check Lynn's vital signs. John dismissed her with a curt nod, then turned to me and smiled, indicating for me to place Lynn on the bed.

As I released her intensely warm body to place her on the bed, her grip tightened and the whimpering became crying.

Wide-eyed, arms folded tightly across her chest, Carol stared at us from the other side of the hospital bed. I could see the moisture coming to her eyes, threatening to overflow onto her cheeks. Abruptly and quickly with a loud sniffle she wiped her teary eyes on the backs of her wrists, then leaned over, placing her hands on the bed.

"It's ok, baby. Mommy is right here..."

With a practiced professionalism, John placed his hands around her waist, and murmured gently to Lynn.

"It's all right, Lynn. Daddy will hold your hand while I see what's going on with your body, ok?"

It took only a few seconds when he said the words I was dreading to hear.

"Rich, I want to do a spinal on your daughter." John said. "We have to rule out meningitis".

My heart felt heavy, as I said, "Okay, do what you have to do."

Carol's expression was hidden by her trembling hands covering her face.

Moving to my wife, I put my arm around her shoulders and held her tightly. Looking down at our daughter I told Lynn, "The doctor needs to do a test, honey. Ok?"

Lynn's fever must have acted like a sedative as she remained anxious, but didn't protest when I said, "Mommy and I will be close by. You're going to be just fine."

We kissed her warm forehead and left the room.

I could hear Dr. Byrd talking to her in low tones as the nurse prepared the instrument tray. I followed the procedure in my mind, as I had seen it many times before. The nurse was curling Lynn into a gentle fetal position on her right side. She held our daughter's her head and knees together to curve her back, which drew the end of her spinal cord up above the level the long spinal would be inserted.

If the needle is inadvertently driven into the spinal cord, all hell breaks loose—searing pain, possible dangerous injury to the cord itself. More likely, the spinal needle bounces off the vertebral bone causing a sharp wince from the patient, and elicits a reassuring response from the physician who is silently biting his lower lip, sensing the sweat flowing down his back, as he re-focuses on keeping a steady hand.

I pictured Dr. Byrd, mask and gloves on, painting a circle of Betadine on Lynn's warm, bare back.

"This will be a little cold, Lynn. Nothing to worry about," I heard him telling Lynn.

I knew what was next, and every muscle on my body tightened in anticipation of my child's scream.

I "saw" Dr. Byrd hold the 3 inch long spinal needle in his right hand, spreading the skin of Lynn's low back between L-3 and L-4, and then he inserted the needle.

Then the scream.

Lynn, my only child, my precious little girl, my angel who trusted me to care for her, protect her, and prevent her from experiencing pain, any pain—-was now in the throes of the worst sensation she has ever experienced in her short time on earth. High-pitched, shrill, and increasing in volume, like a hailstorm of needles blown against soft skin, Lynn's voice penetrated her parents. Carol's cold, damp hands squeezed my hands so hard my knuckles hurt. Our four hands made a sandwich as we bowed our heads, breathed in silence and prayed.

One scream that lasted about two seconds.

Then silence for one more minute.

The door opened and Dr. Byrd had a reassuring smile. "She did just fine. Everything went well. You can go in to see her now."

Partial doctor or not, I was just another slab of humanity called a terrified parent. The tests were negative for meningitis and all Lynn had was a viral infection which resolved in a day or two. But the impact of that moment, the vulnerability and impotence I felt as a father (and later as a patient) has never left me.

PART TWO:

SEPARATION

CHAPTER THIRTEEN

SEE YOU IN SEPTEMBER

". . . . But I have promises to keep,
and miles to go before I sleep,
and miles to go before I sleep."
Robert Frost, *poet*

"See You in September",
The Happenings, 1966

Until that summer, most of my fellow students had been ad-libbing their summers as well; odd jobs, traveling, reading for enjoyment—very little studying. By the end of the third year we had usually chosen an area in medicine of particular interest, one in which we would intern and go on to specialize.

Summer fellowships, often combined with travel, were offered in almost every field. For instance, there was an excellent opportunity to observe advances in a particular type of cancer at a progressive institution and Frank was all over that. Bill took his fellowship at Memorial Hospital in New York, while Toby went to Boston for work in transplantation. Several others went to hospitals in London since their approach to medicine is somewhat different than ours. The British pride themselves on meticulous examination and are less likely to carry out the extensive lab and x-ray studies that we consider routine (because of the money factor, among other things)

At that time, there were two types of fellowships. One stressed academics, providing the student the benefit of great minds and original research in a particular field—lots of conferences and discussions and limited patient responsibility. The other type was more clinical and much less academically oriented. These put the student in a position to assume a great deal of direct patient care.

I chose the second type partly because of its independent nature but mostly because of the unique opportunity that fell in my lap. The resident on my rotation in internal medicine had gone to Harvard Medical School and he raved about a Harvard-sponsored program whereby med students could work at a small Newfoundland hospital. Run by an elderly doctor who had surgical training from the States, this hospital provided early opportunity for surgery otherwise unavailable to me. The juicy cases given to me in Newfoundland were similar to the ones I was "allowed" to do two years later as an intern. The pay was poor—round trip airfare from New York to Gander and the princely sum of $25 a week.

But the fishing was supposed to be great.

Before applying for this long shot opportunity, I discussed it with Carol that night over dinner. Even though it meant a 2 ½ month separation over the summer, our time to be together as a family, my excitement about the professional experience colored my description of the fellowship. Perhaps out of guilt, I down played the possibility of winning it in our conversations. Much to my surprise, Carol enthusiastically encouraged my application…upon reflection, perhaps too enthusiastically.

Our marriage was feeling the strains of the rigors of med school and I had my own doubts about my relationship with Carol.

I didn't want to admit it at first. Maybe it was my long hours, the stress of frequent exams, or competition with my fellow students. Sure, they were all factors in separating me from family life. But the truth of the matter, the real common denominator, was that Carol and I were feeling a slowly growing distance between us. Was it that we were each drifting away equally from our common starting point, that beautiful spring day on Cape Cod when we were married? I think not. Carol was a wonderful mother, a supportive wife and a loving partner. She did nothing to cause me doubt, distraction or heartache. I had to face the cold reality that it was me. I was the one who was losing the love, that close feeling we had for so many years when we lived apart had sustained me with such assurance. Carol was my first girlfriend, my first and only love, and now it was slipping through my fingers like soft sand on Cape Cod.

It bothered me, it confused me, it embarrassed me. Coward that I was, I refused to face it or talk about it. I just let it fester. Apparently she did, too. Rather than a tsunami of arguments increasing in volume and anger, our disintegrating relationship expressed itself as the slow, steady erosion from the tides ebbing and flowing against the beach of our marriage.

My potential job in Newfoundland was not just a unique opportunity—in a very real sense it would be our first separation since we began living together after our marriage, though I think Carol thought it was just a physical one while I perceived it as an emotional one as well. Carol was no dummy, her intellect and intuition was as sharp as it had always been, but she was stoic and kept her emotions to herself.

As luck would have it, Harvard changed its academic schedule so that their students could no longer work there. As I wrote a letter to the hospital requesting the appointment, I realized any hesitation I felt related to not seeing Lynn for the 2 ½ months. The response was an encouraging note requesting letters of recommendation. Soon after that, I was invited to spend the summer there as "extern in surgery". That sure sounded good to me.

When I brought home the good news to Carol, she smiled and congratulated me. Not a word about the separation, or our usual summer plans. Simply a genuine smile before she turned to finish preparing dinner.

I stood there, perhaps a little stunned since I half-way expected a protest, or a question about coming with me, or even if we'd have time to go to the shore before my fourth year started. Lynn must have sensed my confusion because the next thing I knew her arms were wrapped around my knees, and she tugged on my pant leg.

"Up, Daddy, up!"

Our daughter brought me back to the basics: this was definitely a positive professional experience, time well spent, even if it meant a two month separation from my family.

So off I went to Newfoundland, rationalizing my absence as career and relationship enhancing, and who knew? Maybe the result would be good for us.

I packed some old clothes, a couple of medical books, my stethoscope and George Frazer's <u>The Golden Bough.</u> As it turned out, that was the most civilized thing I was to experience all summer. For when I left on Air Canada to the Gander air terminal, I left the normal world, as we know it, far behind.

When I arrived in Gander at 10:30 p.m. June 29, 1966, a note was waiting for me at the deserted ticket office. "Dear Richard—Welcome to Newfoundland! The ferry stops running at midnight so we could never make it back in time. Stay at the local hotel and I will pick you up tomorrow. Look forward to meeting you. Al". Al was the acting director, one of the four doctors who staffed the 92-bed hospital on the tiny island of Twillingate located off the north coast of Newfoundland. Fair enough.

Having the night to myself and my curiosity intact, I looked forward to exploring this new environment. A cab carried me along a pitch black road "to the local hotel, please", and after dumping my heavy suitcase on the almost Victorian bed, I washed up. Water blasted out of the faucets in interrupted and very suggestive spurts, but the rubber plug fit well enough to hold lukewarm water for a quick shave.

I walked downstairs refreshed and looked about the bar. Not what I was expecting exactly, but it was a bar. The bartender was a friendly chap for a Newfie (as the people call themselves) and excused the fact that I was from New York. I decided that it was not the place to ask for a dry martini with a twist, so I asked him to suggest something. Quickly he grabbed a local, musty looking bottle with a screw cap and poured out a clear fluid into a short glass. This was accompanied by a glass of beer which he assured me was a necessary adjunct.

My introduction to the potato based, nearly pure grain product of backwoods soil known as Screech, resulted in hot tears, hotter throat, and a definite flush on my freshly shaven face. "Screech" and there just ain't no other word for it!

I slept well and awoke late. Fortunately, Al was even later.

He was short, round and quiet in his mid-40's, with brown eyes and light brown hair worn a little longer than most of the doctors I knew. Al had a nervous facial tic. Dressed as he was in old khakis, sneakers, and an open shirt, I felt completely out of place with my tie and coat—which I took off at his suggestion and threw in the back seat of his Ford along with my suitcase, never to be put on again.

We headed toward the coast along a dirt and rock road. "This explains my tardiness," he said. "A rock punctured the radiator, and I had had to make periodic stops along the way to refill it. And it took a bit of time to have it fixed in Gander." His apparent nonchalance led me to believe either he was a real loose guy or this type of thing happened often.

An hour later I found out. We stopped to help two men and a woman whose car had gotten a flat with no spare available. It was the damnedest car imaginable—an old gray, worn out Chevy pregnant with supplies, tools and two dogs. It was so loaded down that the fenders almost rested on top of the wheels, and with a flat rear tire the whole thing assumed a pathetic tilt. How they hoped to jack it up was beyond me. And I'm sure they must have had to unload some of it to change the tire. We dropped one of the men off at the nearest village and that was that.

Bright sunshine, large white clouds, and a brisk wind off of the ocean reminded me a lot of the Maine coastline. Inhaling deeply of this fresh salt air brought back memories of other summers on the beach. We turned inland and left the deep blue sea behind us.

Our journey continued, bumping and swerving our way along this monotonous dirt road. The trees were scrawny, wind-whipped by the winter storms. There was no such thing as a row of trees, rather the one or two growing next to each other were almost bent double by the onshore winds. Scrub brush was the only survivor of that harsh environment. Hovering near the ground, the roots gripped the hard earth in a futile effort to avoid the seasonal onslaught. We passed an occasional isolated house, the paint faded to the color of the dirt beneath it. Although still upright, each house looked beaten, lonely and neglected.

God! What a place!

God-forsaken would be more like it.

We finally reached the northern coast of Newfoundland. Fine bits of road dust, like sand paper, pitted my tooth enamel. I ran my tongue over the outer edges of my uppers and wondered what kind of facilities this hospital could possibly have. Even in the summer, the mainland of Newfoundland resembled a sparsely vegetated moonscape. My destination was an island offshore, and I assumed the conditions would have to be worse.

Always up for an adventure, a new experience, an opportunity, a challenge, I assumed I'd always land on my feet...and until then, my assumption was usually justified. Perhaps my Dutch luck had run out...perhaps I had over-estimated the value of this externship on my training...or perhaps I just needed a break from marriage...whatever the reason, I began to think I could have picked a better place for both.

The only way out to the island was a 20 minute ferry ride. It was low tide, which produced a foot-and-a-half gap between the dock and the ferry. Before I could wonder about bridging the gap, Al gunned the engine and began a running start, then neatly jumped the gap without blowing a front tire.

"Best to time your trips with the tides," Al said in his clipped English accent.

I looked at the mainland receding behind us, and then turned to the island we approached. The stark, desolate beauty of this place was like no other coast I had ever seen. The dark green abruptly met jagged, tumbled rocks on the shore. Abundant vegetation in stark contrast with emptiness of the mainland behind us surrounded sturdy evergreens kept low and bent by the vicious winter winds. Inland the trees grew taller and provided employment for men at the Corner Brook paper mill. As we crossed the "tickle" (a narrow stretch of water), I was impressed by the isolation and loneliness on the other side.

Sparsely populated, what kind of people could thrive in this environment? And I wondered about Al, what had made him decide to leave London where he had studied medicine, for such an outpost of medical care. He later told me how much he liked the peace and quiet, but I suspected that his tic might have more accurately reflected his true feelings.

We bumped our way off the ferry and onto the small island that would be my home for the next 10 weeks. The hospital was Spartan. Dirty yellow stucco and weather beaten, it stood out against the sparsely forested background like a discarded shoe box in the grass. No Frank Lloyd Wright influence here.

The steep, cement front steps that led to the clinic had no guardrail, and I was sure that anyone healthy enough to negotiate those steps had to be in pretty good condition. In this clinic, people would call me "doctor" for the first time, and where for the first time they would truly be my patients.

Al introduced me to Mike Keithley, a medical student from St. Bartholomew's Hospital in London. He was a ruddy faced, bubbly, bully-bully sort of a guy. He placed great stock in titles, privileges and what not (both parents were doctors) but in an acceptable way since he was such a jovial fellow. He loved rugby and warm beer and we hit it off well.

Since we were going to be roommates, some ground rules had to be established. He said how he wanted to stay in shape that summer, and would be doing push-ups and sit-ups before breakfast, which he hoped would not disturb me. He didn't do a push-up all summer, smoked a pack a day and didn't bother me at all.

Over supper that first night he told me he intended to enter the field of obstetrics and gynecology, and how much he looked forward to delivering babies. I said that was fine by me, that he could have all the babies if I could have all the appendectomies. We agreed on our preferences and it looked as if things would turn out well. Then he bit into a piece of buttered bread and with an expression of subdued British displeasure, leaned over and quietly said to me, "Careful, Dick, I do believe this is margarine". His royal lips had obviously been used to only the finest of Grade A butter! It promised to be a great summer.

The following Saturday, Mike and I drove the VW van to the very north end of the island, avoiding the rocks and pot holes as best we could. This was our moment of freedom, escaping hospital routine and surveying the Atlantic Ocean from atop the rocky cliffs that fell 400 feet straight down to the ocean. I tested my estimate of height by dropping a rock from the cliff's edge: accelerating at 32 feet per second per second, it took 4 ½ seconds to hit the water- about right. Mike walked over to the nearby light-house, staffed by an old Newfie who had absolutely, hands down, the loneliest job in the world.

They talked for a while and I pulled out a letter from Carol.

I felt lonely too, and sitting there, 400 feet above the vast expanse of the ocean, a bit of nostalgia blew over me. Her letter was newsy, Lynn was having a good summer and starting to read some. I felt a little guilty, pursuing my own interest here in NF, possibly at the expense of my family. It was a feeling that would return.

The rectangular hospital had three floors behind its monotonous façade. Two large wards partially filled the top floor, one for the men and one for the women, each containing 20 steel-framed Florence-Nightingale-type hospital beds with chipped paint. In addition, a very adequate, well equipped OR with non-conductive tile and overhead lamps would be the scene of my first hands-on surgical experience. Three very basic private rooms filled the rest of the floor.

The main floor consisted of a series of smaller adult wards, four to a room, a pediatric ward and the outpatient clinic where minor surgery was performed. An old but very functional x-ray machine sat in a room next to a small lab, the location for basic blood and urine tests.

The "old man's" office was the quintessence of disorganization. Vintage medical texts whose information was obsolete and totally inadequate were scattered around the room. The "old man" was Dr. John Olds, Director of the hospital. He was tall, slender, white haired and extremely terse. He smoked a pipe continuously, spoke in short spurts and rarely smiled. His subdued demeanor indicated difficult times in the past. A board-certified surgeon* who had trained at Johns Hopkins in Baltimore, MD, his parents had guided him into medicine. He was an engineer at heart, and a good one at that. Scattered parts of bony anatomy from various species lay randomly around his office, some half hidden by "Popular Mechanics" or "Journal of the American Medical Association". This room told me as much about his personality as anything I ever experienced that whole summer.

The bottom floor of the hospital contained the laundry room, coal burner, galley and a small room segregated from the rest by a long corridor leading to the coldest part of the building and the morgue. I only went into that room once, the low point of my experience there. Built shortly after World War I, without central heating or electricity, the hospital now boasted its own independent generator system which sat up on the hill behind the building.

---

* A Board Certified surgeon has been fully trained in an approved residency program, taking up to five years for a general surgeon, during which time he/she has amassed experience as primary surgeon in a significant number of operations, operations of all types: routine, challenging, cancer involved, trauma related. For this he receives a diploma, which allows him the privilege to apply for a grueling written exam which, if he passes, allows him the further privilege to apply for a grueling oral exam which, if he again passes, allows him to be called a "Board Certified Surgeon". He is ready for the world! Keep in mind that he graduated from high school 14 years earlier! Board Certification means the highest level of professionalism in each of the medical specialties.

Powered by coal delivered twice a month, guess who was assigned the shovel? There's nothing like moving tons of coal from flat boat to storage to keep in shape. Most of the island, whose 3,000 inhabitants lived off the fertile sea, was without telephone service or electricity. Oil lamps and cast iron wood-burning stoves provided light and heat.

Several nearby islands shared the medical facility in Twillingate. Patients arrived by seaworthy craft of various descriptions, in all kinds of weather. In spite of its geographic isolation, the hospital was very active and the surgical schedule full and varied.

In the pre-isoniazed and streptomycin days (antibiotics used for treatment of TB after the 1940's), the old man had saved many a TB victim's life by removing the infected lung. His reputation grew with each patient, and people continued to travel miles across the timberland and waterways of Newfoundland to be treated by "Dr. John". The cases that I assisted on included gastrectomy for cancer of the stomach, pyloroplasty and vagotomy for duodenal ulcer, pyloromyotomy for pyloric stenosis, laminectomy, prostatectomy, laparotomy, removal of a huge ovarian cyst weighing 9 pounds, hysterectomy, tonsillectomies and appendectomies.

To be first assistant on such cases, let alone performing an appendectomy myself, was a privilege I didn't have again until I was an intern a year and a half later.

The doctors were paid a fixed salary by the government and medical care was entirely subsidized. A man paid $6 a year for himself, $10.50 for his entire family. That entitled him to all medical privileges—outpatient visits, medications, in hospital care, surgery, deliveries and pediatric care. This was an economic necessity for a people whose average yearly income was under $700. Unfortunately, things such as canned food, fresh fruit and meat, which had to be shipped long distances, were very expensive and considered luxuries. Most inhabitants rarely supplemented their parochial seafood diet with those items.

Newfoundland was part of the Grand Banks region, with abundant seafood of every variety, especially cod. Fish were caught in the spring and summer either with nets or by jigging. The nets were tough nylon and the fish would entangle their fins in the fine meshwork trying to fight their way out. In the morning the men would pull the nets in, hand over hand, and pick off the wiggling fish like ornaments off of a Christmas tree.

"Jigging" fascinated me. The men drifted about in their dories up to a mile offshore and would drop a weighted hook down several fathoms. Every five to six seconds they would sharply yank on the line (jig the line) three or four feet, and then let the hook drift down again. The fast movement of the flashing hook attracted the fish, and eventually one would get hooked through the stomach, back or fin and then be pulled to the surface. Imagine how abundant the fish had to be for jigging to be successful!

The fish were split open and cleaned, then flattened out on wooden jetties to dry in the sun. Each fisherman had his own jetty which projected out into the water 50 feet, a small shack at the end. The dried fish were stored in tall neat piles in the shack, each layer of fish separated by a thick covering of rock salt. The salted cod were then placed in underground sheds for consumption during the sparse winter months. The amount of salt consumed by the inhabitants of Twillingate was extremely high, and I became interested in the correlation between salt consumption and the high prevalence of hypertension on the island and in similar communities.

Salt cannot build up in the bloodstream above a certain concentration because of potential harmful effects. So as a defensive mechanism to high salt intake, the body will conserve water to help dilute the salt to acceptable body levels. The additional volume of water must find room in the bloodstream, thus contributing to elevated blood pressure. Consequently, people with a history of hypertension are placed on a low salt diet in an attempt to alleviate their condition.

It seemed like a unique opportunity to investigate this correlation, and I did a study on this subject by interviewing and examining patients, going over hospital records and comparing patient histories. I started groups of patients on various anti-hypertensive regimens and compared the results over the course of the summer. I had my own hypertensive clinic, something unheard of for a fourth year med student at a university center. I don't know if I did much good in my short time in Twillingate. Dr. John had correctly identified the high salt intake as the culprit and was not sanguine about the long term benefits of my undertaking. However, he gave me the independence to pursue this effort.

This study also served as the basis for my term thesis. All medical students at the University of Rochester had to submit a thesis prior to graduation. Some got theirs in just under the wire on the eve of graduation which plagued their last sublime days as students. My experience on paper was less painful; however, what it led up to was losing my patient.

Even though most of the hypertensive population seemed to peacefully coexist with their silent enemy, there were tragic exceptions. For instance, Peter Darcey, a 37 year-old fisherman, father of three, and never sick a day in his life, came to the clinic complaining of a pounding headache. Dirty blond hair shoved under a dark blue watch cap, Peter had a history of mild, intermittent headaches in the past.

That day was the big day for the community fishermen: the lobster and cod catch. So vital to his and the community's financial survival, this annual catch was the make-it or break-it event that marked the entire season. For Peter to appear in the clinic rather than on his boat, indicated the severity of his pain. Newfies are stoics. A product of harsh weather, limited resources, and a stubborn resignation about their survival, the typical resident never complained about anything. For Peter to seek medical help on the most important day of his professional year clearly communicated the seriousness of his ailment; his presence in my office on that particular day told me more than his words did about the severity of his pain and the gravity of his ailment.

After arriving in my office looking as if a meat cleaver was bisecting his skull he readily admitted taking up to 10 aspirin a day, a potentially toxic dose that could cause bleeding. By then I knew enough to not chastise him for waiting so long to see me.

Wincing from the pain in his head, Peter was slumped over on the examination table. His watch cap in his hands, he nervously rotated it as I reviewed his chart. His blood pressure jumped out at me: 220/110! Normal blood pressure is 140/80 or less. The first number, or systolic pressure, represents 140 millimeters of mercury, the maximum pressure inside the arteries when the heart squeezes. Take a garden hose and close off the nozzle. Now turn on the faucet and watch the hose expand under pressure—that's the systolic pressure. Now turn the faucet off and the hose collapses—that lower pressure is called the diastolic pressure and represents the arterial pressure in between heartbeats.

Obviously, Peter's blood pressure was dangerously high. I stressed the importance of decreasing his salt intake (not a practical suggestion in Twillingate where in the absence of electricity, fish can be preserved only in salt). When I handed him the little white pills, I emphasized the importance of taking BP medication not only to relieve his pain, but also to maintain his health. Apparently, my words failed to penetrate the pain of his headache beyond their assurance of long term relief. All Peter cared about was getting rid of his headache pronto. But formal medical care and prescription drugs were considered options of the last resort by most Newfies. Unfortunately, he neglected the BP meds . . .Instead, he upped his aspirin and suddenly died of a massive stroke, probably due to a cerebral hemorrhage. I was devastated since I felt responsible. Maybe I hadn't explained it adequately. I was filled with self doubt and guilt. Now a family of 5 was a family of 4 with no father. I felt as if I was practicing in the dark ages and I saw, first hand, the danger of assuming I had communicated effectively. This was the first death for which I felt true responsibility—not an easy reality to digest. It would not be the last.

CHAPTER FOURTEEN

THE OLD MAN

"Leaders are visionaries with a poorly developed sense of fear and no concept of the odds against them. They make the impossible happen."
Robert Jarvik, inventor of the first artificial heart

"Hit the road Jack, and don't you come back no more, no more, no more..."
"Hit the Road Jack", Ray Charles, 1961

The morning of my first experience in this Spartan, generator driven operating room, I awoke early and quietly shaved while Mike, who had forgotten to get up for his celebrated push-ups, slept peacefully on. I went down for a small breakfast of tea and a hard roll which sat like a rock in the pit of my stomach.

I briefly stepped outside the hospital which gave me time to quell my performance anxiety, and allow the fresh air to blow away any doubts that arose to distract me from meeting the challenge awaiting me in the OR.

At precisely 8 o'clock I met Al in the OR.

What a tingle! Here I was masquerading as an intern, yet I was only a lowly third year med student. Was I up to the challenge? You bet. As Braer Rabbit said, "Just throw me into the brier patch". I wasn't distracted by a flock of other "doe-in-the-headlights" med students, all trying to look smart but not knowing diddly about the OR. It was just me, the Old Man, the Filipina scrub nurse and Al "passing gas". I mean, I was the co-pilot in the room, never having flown a plane before. On the other hand, I had to control my excitement since I didn't know diddley either. Iron man had nothing on me!

While Mike was seeing clinic patients, I was going to assist on my first operation—a cholecystectomy (gall bladder removal). While the patient was being anesthetized, I changed into my greens taking extra care to tuck my shirt into my pants. The last action was shoving the drawstring behind the waist band in order to avoid contaminating the field from any of my clothing.

Many anesthetic agents are potential hazards because of their explosive nature, so I wore non-conductive OR shoes. At this point, the Old Man appeared on the scene. He was in his greens, a tall thin figure whose weathered, tan face contrasted with puffs of white hair showing beneath his surgical cap. His hands were shoved into the front of his pants and his mask was undone and fell against his chest. This in itself was a mild breach of sterile precautions, but nothing compared with the pipe stuck in his mouth. I was sure it wasn't lit because of the anesthetic gas hazard, but the dried ashes could easily blow out and float about in the air. I was appalled to see how wrong I was when he sucked in a mouthful of thick smoke just as Al introduced us.

I didn't know whether to scramble for cover or maintain my cool and shake his hand. The Old Man saved me from both by leaving the room after an acknowledging nod and mumbled something like, "I hope you've worked on a gall bag before."

"Yes sir!" I lied.

His hope was unjustified, but I told him I had because I didn't want to lose the opportunity to assist. The nurses helped the patient, a 42 year-old male, on to the OR table. Next they placed a blood pressure cuff onto his left upper arm which was supported on an arm board. A rubber tourniquet was applied to his right biceps and a large vein swelled up over his right forearm. An 18-gauge needle inserted into the vein allowed a rush of dark blood into the attached syringe. The tourniquet was removed, the syringe detached, and IV tubing was connected to the needle and secured in place with white surgical tape. The glass bottle dripped, drip, dripped its saline solution through the IV tubing into the vein, flushing the red-tinged fluid clear (today all IV fluids are contained in plastic bags; they're cheaper, lighter and don't shatter when accidentally dropped onto the floor).

The hospital pediatrician had been recruited as anesthesiologist, and he was competent with his previous OJT (on the job training) instead of formal training. He placed the oxygen mask over the patient's nose and mouth, and after a few reassuring words, he administered a short-acting Phenobarbital IV to induce rapid onset of sleep while he bled in general anesthetic gas via the mask to keep the patient under.

Then he added a muscle relaxant (succinyl choline at that time). Although classified as a muscle relaxant, succinyl choline and similar substances, when given in sufficient dosage, act as paralytic agents, albeit it temporarily, since they render all voluntary muscles (not the heart) totally non-functional.

In fact, these two drugs are currently the first two of three drugs administered in lethal injections—phenobarbital puts the condemned asleep and the profound muscle relaxant prevents the person from breathing since all muscles of respiration are paralyzed. During surgery the anesthesiologist* does the breathing for you—not to worry. The third drug is a high concentration of potassium which stops the heart by preventing sodium-potassium exchange across the muscle cell wall, thus shutting down muscle contraction.

The Old Man scrubbed up. Hands are always held above the elbows so water and soap slide from clean to dirty (hands to elbows). Scrubbing starts with a special soft brush impregnated with soap or Betadine. First, we scrub the fingers and hands, and then move circumferentially around the wrists and forearms. We discard the brush and thoroughly rinse, again from the hands to the elbows to allow all contamination to flow into the sink.

Our hands held forward and above the elbows, the Old Man entered the OR. The nurse handed him a sterile towel. Then he dried off, starting at his fingers and hands, working down his forearms to the elbows, and then discarded the towel.

The scrub nurse fitted us with sterile gowns and gloves. The Old Man slipped smoothly into his gloves. It's not as easy as it looks, and rather embarrassing when

---

*The joke that all surgeons love to tell: "Question—What is the definition of an anesthesiologist? Answer—someone half awake trying to keep someone else (the patient) half asleep".

you cram one of your fingers awkwardly into the wrong slot.

Trying to emulate the Old Man with the ease in which he inserted his fingers into the appropriate slots, all I managed to do was cram index and middle finger into the thumb, pull out, and try again where the thumb slid in perfectly, as did the index finger. If those were the only two fingers I had, all would have been well; however, the two middle fingers decided to mate in the third slot, leaving my pinkie curled painfully in the palm.

I felt flop sweat beading on my forehead. I glanced at the nurse staring down at my hands. If she was hiding a smirk behind her mask, her eyes didn't indicate it. Taking a deep breath, I withdrew my hands slightly and tried again. This time it worked. With great relief, I took my assigned spot beside the operating table.

The nurse started to prep the exposure of white abdominal flesh with gauze soaked in white Phisohex surgical soap. The incision would be just below the right costal margin (ribs) and she started in a circular pattern, scrubbing from the center and working outward; then with new gauze started over at the proposed sight of surgery and worked out again. The principle is always to prep from clean area to unsterile area, never the opposite.

Sterile water washed the soap away, and the incision site was draped with sterile towels and sheets. The Old Man stepped up to the table, pipe gone and mask in place, took the scalpel and made a quick, clean incision which carried through the skin and fat down to the muscle layer in one swift, sure motion. Almost as a delayed reaction, rich bright red blood filled the trough where the knife had passed as if the wound took a moment to respond. No backwoods surgeon, this one—he knew exactly what to do, and did it aggressively.

The abdominal wall has seven layers: skin (epidermis and dermis), subcutaneous tissue (varies from less than ½ inch of fat to greater than 6 inches in obese individuals), a thin layer of fibrous tissue called Scarpa's fascia, the thick gristle-like fascia layer that covers and protects the muscle, and finally the delicate saran wrap-like covering of the abdominal cavity called the peritoneum.

The thicker the fat layer, the greater the challenge is to the surgeon. Fat generally does not bleed much, but can be troublesome during an operation because it takes more effort to retract an abdominal wall that is 8 inches thick. It is the assistant's obligation to keep the abdominal wall away from the surgeon's work space; and the thicker the abdominal wall, the more tiresome it is to maintain the separation...especially during a prolonged surgery. (Currently, large oval steel bars with attached retractors are used to free the assistant for more useful work).

Post-operatively, fat increases the risk of a variety of complications. Fat provides a perfect medium for bacteria to grow. Translation—obesity lends itself to a much higher rate of post-operative wound infections, which may result in total wound disruption, or dehiscence, where intestines bubble up through the open wound and end up lying on the skin. (Dehiscence is more likely to occur in obese persons even in the absence of wound infection).

Several post-operative respiratory complications are also associated with obesity. The recovering, recumbent patient has much more difficulty breathing against a wall of fat. In the erect or standing position the diaphragm is aided by gravity in its descent during inspiration. In the recumbent position the diaphragm's descent is hindered by the not insignificant weight of fat pressing down on the abdomen. The diaphragm must compete for space with the patient's excess fat.   Occasional deep breaths keep the lungs inflated and reduce the risk of pneumonia.   Deep breathing is more difficult for obese persons and thus they have a greater risk of collapse of focal segments of lung tissue (called atelectasis) and resultant pneumonia.   Finally, they have an increased risk of reflux of gastric juices and aspiration of such juices and saliva into the lungs, resulting in aspiration pneumonia.   Consequently, post-op orders require the nurses to maintain the obese patient in a semi-sitting position with the head of the bed at a 45 degree angle.   This facilitates breathing, since the lungs are not battling against a diaphragmatic barricade buttressed by a wall of fat lurking inside the abdomen.   Instead, gravity tends to equalize the playing field, forcing the intra-abdominal fatty bucket to descend towards the pelvis, allowing greater space in the upper abdomen for the diaphragm to descend and the lungs to expand.

My job was to retract and suction, keeping my hands the hell out of the abdomen, and "...to do no harm".

Fortunately our patient was slender and had offered no impediment to the Old Man's swift incision—down through the dermis, subcutaneous tissue and Scarpa's fascia in one motion. There lay the glistening fascial layer covering muscle, both of which were carefully incised. Bleeding was controlled by clamping and tying the culprit blood vessels with silk ties (nowadays cautery is usually used to seal off bleeding vessels). The thin peritoneum was divided and suddenly the entire contents of the abdominal cavity came into dramatic view. The old man pointed the tips of his forceps.

"What's that, Richard?"

"Omentum".

"And that?"

"Transverse colon".

"What's this?"

"Common duct."

"And this?"

"Cystic duct."

"And that?"

"Duodenum".

So far, so good.

Just don't ask me how to take out the gallbladder.

"What's the first instrument I need to take out the gallbladder?"

Uhhhhhhhhh....my mind went blank.

The nurse saved my bacon by handing him a large curved Kelly clamp.

"K-kelly clamp!" I said too late, and too loudly as the Old Man grasped the tip of the gallbladder and pulled gently.

"Follow along with me and help me isolate the cystic duct."

Like a fuzzy picture snapping into focus, my eyes zoomed in on the clamp and the greenish avocado shaped gall bladder attached by the cystic duct to the inch-long common bile duct which drains into the small intestine. Steady hands followed the Old Man's directions with a determination that previously I had only hoped I possessed—-and now I knew the assurance, the confidence, and yes, the skill I had seen demonstrated by others was mine for the taking.

"Good. Now take the long right angle clamp and pass it under the cystic duct. I'll feed you the 2-0 silk tie, grab it with the right angle and tie off the cystic duct. Use 3 tight square knots".

I felt like saying, "Aye, aye, sir!" and clicking my heels. Instead, I did as I was told——grateful for the opportunity to do it.

Holy shit! This is fun! I love it!

"Cut the suture just above the knot."

Years later during internship, the maligning Chief Resident would always criticize us for cutting the suture either too long or too short. The last day on the service a ballsy intern asked the Chief, "How do you want me to cut the suture—too long or too short?"

The Old Man didn't say anything so I guess I cut it correctly. We tied off the cystic duct again and cut the duct between the two ties. We did the same for the cystic artery and removed the gallbladder from its bed nestled against the liver. We checked for bleeding, removed the lap pads and closed the abdomen in three layers: heavy suture material for the deep fascia, above and below the muscle layer, and smaller suture material for the skin closure. Interestingly, the divided muscle is not sutured since it does not have the integrity to hold a snuggly tied suture and will only pull part on contraction. Fortunately, the muscle heals to itself, and remarkably with no loss of strength. So ended my first gallbladder operation.

My admiration for the Old man soared. He was always self-assured and confident, and always demanded definitive criteria and clear indications for his every action. Like Opa's knowledge and talent with cams, nuts, bolts, calipers, lathes, welders, and grinders, Dr. John's precision and instinct never failed him during my summer of observation and education.

At times I would politely challenge his approach on the basis of largely theoretical knowledge that I had acquired so far in med school, and he would encourage me to prove myself right or wrong by assessing what actually happens in clinical practice. Feeling rebuffed, and a little patronized, I kept my pouting to myself and continued to query my mentor whenever I felt it appropriate.

At first I mistook his rigidity as being too narrow, yet he had based his approach on a synthesis of his medical experiences. He had chosen those practices and procedures that he had found to work, and adopted patterns of care that achieved the best results. He encouraged me to do the same.

"Richard, the longest walk for a surgeon is from one side of the OR table (the assisting side) to the other (the surgeon's side)." He said this with what passed for a smile on his narrow face.

Every interaction with the Old Man was an experience. Yes, he was good with his hands. Very good. It all fit, I suppose—a highly intelligent, well-trained, extremely reticent man isolated in a very desolate environment. Unfortunately, I never got to know much of the Old Man's life, past or present. But I learned some of the structure of that man, enough to piece him together though in a more static than dynamic sense, for I could never figure out what he really wanted or where he was headed. His previous wife had died and no one knew the circumstances as he never mentioned her. He had remarried a local woman, and I never met her nor did I ever hear him speak of her.

There was a respectful reticence about Dr. John throughout the island, as if undue curiosity about the man's past was an affront to his presence. Everyone's privacy was respected, but Dr. John's position in the community guaranteed a loyal silence from the other inhabitants on the island.

One night, over dinner, Al told me all he knew about the "Old Man".

A graduate of Johns Hopkins University in Baltimore, Maryland, he had wanted to go into engineering. His courses and manual talents all pointed in that direction. At his mother's insistence he entered medicine instead. How she managed this and what concessions he had made and what resentments he might have held are only speculative. Nevertheless, he completed medical school and went on to become a well-trained and accredited general surgeon. About 1938 he migrated from the U.S. to this little outpost of Newfoundland.

He was instrumental in converting the existing building into a workable, well-equipped and electrically powered, centrally heated hospital that could provide medical services in a significant way. One room in the basement of the hospital was his workshop. It bore a close resemblance to his office and it reminded me of a blacksmith's shop. It was filled with machines for metal work mostly—drill set, lathe, lock saws, welding torch, scraps of rusted iron, unlabelled oil cans, an old tractor engine and so on. He had built some exquisite and practical things for his house, and was the fix-it man when anything mechanically too difficult for the janitor presented itself.

A perfect example of the Old Man and his island was his ability to provide a prosthetic leg for a child whose leg he was forced to amputate as the result of an infection.

The island society was not genetically diverse. Families were not large in general, but they continued to remain there generation after generation, so it was inevitable that cousin would marry cousin, increasing the likelihood that recessive genes would be manifested. Every trait in a person, such as blue eyes, blonde hair and height is controlled by the genes received from both parents. These genes may be either recessive, in which case they won't be manifested in a person's appearance unless that person receives a recessive gene from each parent, or dominant, in which case they will be manifested, even if a person receives both a dominant and recessive gene.

In other words, inheritance of both a recessive and dominant gene for the same trait will result in expression of only the dominant gene. The recessive gene trait will be expressed only in the presence of inheritance of both recessive genes. If a man carries a recessive gene that results in a defective blood clotting factor, it will not affect him since it is recessive, and it will not affect his children for the same reason. However, if his wife has, by some rare chance, the same recessive gene then each parent may pass this gene onto a child. If that child receives two recessive genes, it will develop a bleeding problem. The chances are much greater that both parents will carry such a recessive gene if they are related through common grandparents, i.e. are cousins.

Thus, in a relatively static society, genetic defects have a greater chance of becoming manifest. And that is exactly what happened on this tiny little island off the coast of Newfoundland. One family on the island was cultivating its own inherited bleeding problem, and family members had to be extremely careful—a fairly difficult task in an active fishing community where knives and fishhooks are a common hazard. Eventually, the inevitable happened. A 3 year-old boy had cut his leg on an axe and they could not stop the bleeding. Blood for transfusion was unavailable and tourniquets were applied. The bleeding stopped but the leg became badly infected and had to be amputated. He recovered and showed a persistent desire to stand up and walk despite his handicap. The Old Man designed and made a small artificial leg from material in his workshop. It was a bit cumbersome and heavy but it never held back the determination of that 3 year-old boy.

Stories like this were sounding a bit apocryphal to me until a patient entered the hospital and presented a problem which demanded the mechanical skill of the Old Man. The patient's name was Joe—a huge, very overweight, white haired, barrel-chested, tight lipped Newfie who had been one of the Old Man's friends for a long time. Joe was a two-pack-a-day smoker and always had a hacking cough. Recently the cough had gotten worse and his voice slightly hoarse. When I examined him in the clinic, his chest was full of wheezes. His x-ray showed a suspicious shadow on the right side near the main bronchus. I admitted him to the hospital that same afternoon. The Old Man came by to see Joe after the x-ray and told him he wanted to keep him there to do a few tests. I knew what that meant and left the patient's room before he could read his future on my face. Joe was in for a long, tough struggle to survive.

Joe's daughter Joan was the head nurse at the hospital. She was really a great gal—smart, a strapping sort, stable as a rock and married to one of the few locals interested in higher education (A degree at the University of St. John's was in his future). Joe was my patient while he was in the hospital, and Joan and her husband often invited me over for some tea and good laughs. She, of course, was very concerned about her father and we would discuss him occasionally, but she was too much of a realist to have false hopes. From my perspective, one of the most fulfilling aspects of medicine has been the depth of communication that I pride myself in having with family members concerning the stricken patient, modern HIPPA (Health Insurance Portability and Accountability Act which regulates confidentiality of patient identification and records) regulations notwithstanding.

Eventually Joe started to spit up blood and his breathing became progressively worse. We had to bring in an oxygen tank and Joe would sit on the edge of his sagging, old steel-spring hospital bed puffing and sweating and sucking air from the mask on which he was becoming more and more dependent every day. We wanted to perform a bronchoscopy to determine the cause of his bleeding. At that time, this procedure was performed with a rigid bronchoscope, a long straight tube with a light source to visualize the main branches of the bronchial tree as the tube is inserted through the mouth and into the trachea with the patient completely sedated. The hospital had no such instrument, an expensive item whose limited use in this hospital could not justify the cost. So the Old Man retired to his workshop and constructed a functional bronchoscope from a small pipe and the light source from a sigmoidoscope. Ingenious and it worked. Unfortunately, it confirmed the cancer we suspected and could do nothing about.

Joe was in one of the few semi-private rooms, partly because of the nature of his illness, which required frequent nursing attention and bulky oxygen equipment, but mostly because the Old Man wanted this for his close friend. Joe's roommate, Danny, was a strong, wiry typically reticent elderly Newfie who had developed a simple case of pneumonia and was too weak to be treated at home. I admitted him to the hospital and gave him procaine penicillin 1.2 million units intra-muscular injections each day for 4 days.

I had him cough deeply the first day in order to produce sputum that I could examine under the microscope. In larger hospitals the sputum would be sent in a sterile jar to a lab to culture it on special nutrient plates and report in two days the exact type of bacteria involved, and the drugs it was sensitive to. Small round discs, each containing a single antibiotic, are placed among the colonies. The discs that contained the effective antibiotic for that particular bacterial colony will inhibit its growth and leave a clear spot on the culture medium. We didn't have culture plates so I used a microscope to try to identify the bacteria causing Danny's pneumonia.

The slide was loaded with white blood cells and blue stained, round, paired bacteria, typical of pneumococci bacteria, which in that era were very sensitive to penicillin.

He responded well and in several days he was walking around the room pestering me to let him go home.

Like most Newfies, he thought hospitals were houses of death, and he had never been in one before. Though he never discussed it, it was apparent that the entire experience frightened him. Reminding him of his own mortality, Danny's awareness of Joe's condition did not help his situation. He was so grateful with his reprieve that he offered me the use of a dory and several lobster pots.

The following week Mike and I purchased lobster licenses from the local fish warden for 25 cents each. One sunny blustery day, after 5 o'clock rounds, we went down to Danny's jetty. His broad smile greeted us and he spent a few minutes explaining where to place the pots and how to catch bait. We must have appeared helpless for he told us to get into the dory and then he hopped in himself. I rowed quietly along the water's edge. The depth was about 8 feet, and the tide was rolling in beneath a smooth sea.

Standing on the shore side of the dory, balancing on steady feet in thick soled boots, Danny lifted a 12 foot pole with a blunt barbed prong on the end, and slipped it softly into the water. Then with a quick stroke, he drove it deep into the dark blue water. Just as quickly he pulled it back and up and out of the water. Impaled on the prong squirmed a large, beautiful flounder. Danny shook it onto the floor of the boat and cut into it with a swift slice of his knife. Each half went into a lobster pot and we were ready to set the traps.

It was almost a shame to use the succulent, fat flounder for lobster bait, and I asked him to spear another so we could have it for supper. He looked at me in reserved disgust. Newfies never eat anything that serves as bait. This unspoken tradition caused the waste of a lot of good food. I swear that if they could use lobsters to catch some lobster-eating fish, they would never eat lobster again. Whenever possible, Mike and I ignored this custom, but only in secrecy so as not to insult our Newfie neighbors.

Apparently, we passed Danny's seaworthy test so the dory was available for us every day at sunset. We would take the VW bus down to the dory and shove off to check the pots. When we didn't get a lobster we speared a floun-der. We ate well, and it was as much the excitement of catching it ourselves, as it was the freshness of the seafood that made it taste so good.

Interestingly, flounder and lobster have very similar camouflage markings. The disc shaped flounder is dark brown with small white spots, and lies quietly on the bot-tom to feed on smaller fish called capelin. They are very difficult to see unless you are a Newfie, but over the sum-mer we developed Newfie eyes. Underneath, by contrast, they are pure white, which seems in defiance of the princi-ple of camouflage; however it makes them blend with the sky when seen from below.

The first day out, when I pulled up the lobster pot, all I could see was the barnacle encrusted, seaweed covered, drip-ping wet wood slot framework of the trap with the flounder's white belly showing inside the inverted net cone. After unhinging the trap, I stuck my hand in to adjust the bait and then I saw the antennae and black eyes of a Newfie lobster. The chitinous covering was typically dark green speckled with dark black, but underneath she was overflowing with bright orange eggs. We threw her back into the water. It was early July and this was bound to happen, but our first catch had been logged and more were to come.

CHAPTER FIFTEEN

GOODBYE JOE

"No man is an island...."
John Donne, poet
(even when he's on one)

"Never My Love", The Association, 1965

As the summer flew by, thoughts of Carol and Lynn intruded and confused me in my rare moments of solitude. There were no public phones on the island, and in those days, long distance and especially international long distance was prohibitively expensive. So we communicated by mail.

After four years of marriage, it was strange not to climb into bed with my wife. Instead, I had to endure an Englishman snoring on the other side of the room. I missed the comforts of home, the love from my little girl who thought her daddy was just the greatest and Carol's home cooking. And I did miss Carol. But I did not feel the intensity of love that I once had, and that bothered me. I did not mention my ambivalence when I wrote which was only on occasion. I stuck to the facts and details of my day, trying to relate my excitement about the opportunity and my observations of the culture on this island outpost——a far cry from any experience either Carol or I had ever had.

Carol and Lynn spent these weeks in Rochester following the routine we had established during the school year. Carol had her work; Lynn had her day care, so the only change was my 24 hour absence for those ten weeks. Her letters were similar in tone, content and frequency—newsy and informative about their lives at home. Carol's letters were pleasant, but further evidence that the distance between us had become more than just the miles between us. I vaguely remembered the passion each of us put in the letters we had exchanged in boarding school and the early years of college. My letters expressed my enthusiasm for everything I was learning, my appreciation for the hardiness of the people who came to the clinic, and the stark contrast between my urban medical education and this rural medical experience.

> *"Success is the ability to go from one fail-ure to another with no loss of enthusiasm."*
> *Winston Churchill, English Prime Minister*

I heard the familiar sound of Joe's cough as I walked down the hallway toward his room. The Old Man's friend had been following a progressive downhill course, but in the last two days he said he actually felt better. He had stopped coughing blood and his breathing had improved. He was eating breakfast so I had a quick listen to his lungs and scooted off to the OR.

The first case was a tonsillectomy on a 6 year-old girl and I was hoping the Old Man would let me do part of it. The patient was asleep and I was in my greens, scrubbed and ready to assist. At this point the Old Man, dressed in civilian clothes, poked his head through the OR door and asked if I had ever done a tonsillectomy before.

"No, sir." I said.

"Then I'd better stick around." That was the understatement of the day.

I persuaded him to scrub in and guide my shaking hands. Fifty-five minutes and many heartbeats later I sewed up the tonsil bed and was never more relieved to be through with a case.

A tonsillectomy is much harder to do than an appendectomy. There is only so much room in a person's mouth, and not enough room for more than one surgeon. Definitely not a team effort. Also, the very large and very important carotid artery is deep in the tonsillar bed. After the tonsil is snipped and removed this bed must be sutured together. If the needle passes too deeply it will pierce the artery and all hell breaks loose. I knew all of the potential hazards. What I didn't know was how to remove tonsils. Perhaps my sweat beaded brow indicated my anxiety, and for once the Old Man was patient. I somehow survived the operation.

Oh, and my patient survived as well.

That afternoon I went to check on her in the pediatric ward where she was sleeping. The nurse said she had vomited blood once but otherwise was doing well. The sight of this innocent child reminded me of my own daughter so far away in New York. I checked her chart again to make sure her vitals were where they were supposed to be so soon after surgery.

In an adjacent crib was a 3 week-old baby whom I hadn't seen before. Black hair in curls over her dainty ears, the baby girl lay on her side and was peacefully asleep. The nurse said she had just been admitted because of persistent vomiting after meals over the last 5 days. I checked the chart, but in his typical fashion the old man had scribbled only a few words at the bottom of the sheet—"admit for observation—vomiting." Dr. John rarely put down more information than this, so I contacted her mother to get the full story.

Her mother had the same dark hair and healthy ruddy complexion as her daughter. She told me her daughter weighed 8 lbs. 2 oz. at birth and had nursed well for the first week of her life. However, she had started vomiting occasionally the following week, usually after feedings. Her mother twisted a loose lock of her own dark hair as she told me about her daughter's vomiting with every meal. Now her weight was down to 7 lbs. 8 oz. Knowing that was not unusual (many babies drop a few ounces after birth) I nevertheless thought this sounded like pyloric stenosis, a congenital blockage of the short canal between the stomach and the small intestine.

I caught up with the Old Man on his way back to his office and discussed my concern and "professional" opinion with his disappearing back. He stopped short, almost causing me to flop into him, before turning around to face me. A slight smile accompanied his assurance that infantile vomiting occurred more often than not, and this was most likely not pyloric stenosis but something more common, such as colic.

"The bird on the lawn is a sparrow, not a canary," is a British medical saying indicating common things happen commonly. For the time being, I would accept the Old Man's sparrow.

The Old Man gave me another patient, an elderly man who was very upset about being hospitalized. The heart and electrocardiograms fascinated me, so I had brought a book with me to Newfoundland on interpretations of EKGs (the tracings of the electrical activity of the heart). Having recently completed an excellent course in cardiology, I had a lot of fresh information in my mind.

As soon as a patient with a cardiac problem came into the hospital, I would be there with the EKG machine. One of the few things the Old Man knew very little about, he called me to help interpret a tracing. What an ego boost! My early success was a 46 year-old man with left anterior chest pain that came on with exercise or eating, and disappeared with rest. I took pre and post-exercise EKGs and pointed out changes in the post-exercise S-T segment indicative of heart strain, or ischemia (inadequate blood flow to the cardiac muscle tissue). Of course the history was suggestive of angina, but it was gratifying to confirm it on the EKG strip and diagnose it myself. Based on these findings, I put him on nitroglycerine, which alleviated the chest pain.

My inherited cardiac patient had developed progressive shortness of breath over the last few months, plus ankle swelling in late afternoon, and had to sleep upright with two pillows so he could get up to urinate 2 or 3 times each night. Examination revealed an irregular pulse and an enlarged heart, confirmed by chest x-ray. The EKG showed evidence of heart strain, enlarged left ventricle and atrial fibrillation, which caused the irregular pulse. The underlying cause of his condition was arterioscleroisis of the coronary arteries, which resulted in the heart muscle not getting proper nourishment and therefore slowly failing. I felt that he should receive digitalis to assist his weak heart and checked his chart to see what the Old Man suggested. "Admit" in the Old Man's scribble was the only word on the page.

Starting a patient on digitalis for the first time must be done gradually and carefully so as to avoid giving too much of the drug and thereby causing a variety of potentially serious side effects. Digitalis can present problems…even for the experienced cardiologist, and I wasn't about to start administering digitalis on my own. I phoned Dr. John and told him I thought our patient needed digitalis.

"Yup. Suspect he does." I heard a draw on his ever present pipe." How's your post-op tonsillectomy doing?"

"What?" Jerked back to the reality of being in charge of more than one person in the hospital that night, I replied. "Oh, she's doing very well."

"Check her again later tonight," and he hung up.

Back to my medical book. The familiar text on the relevant page suddenly began to dance across the page; jump, jive, do-si-do and finally settle into a familiar fox trot as my mind re-absorbed the information. I took notes and wrote down dosages. One of the guidelines in digitalizing a patient is to follow the day-to-day EKG pattern which will show a change in the S-T segment at the optimal dosage. So with a brave heart and queasy stomach accompanying an uneasy feeling of undeserved responsibility, I wrote down my orders in the nurse's book. Until then I must have taken his pulse 5 times a day to assure myself he wasn't going to die because of an error—a wrong dose—on my part.

He had survived the initial dose.

He complained that he wanted to go home.

He had survived the first day.

I calculated, re-calculated, checked and re-checked my information prior to writing the order for the second dose.

He complained more loudly that he wanted to go home.

He had survived the second day.

More calculations, more checks, more re-checks all yielding the same information.

Another day and another increase in the dose. I no longer heard his complaints, nor the loudness of his voice asserting them, as I held my breath and took his pulse. On the third day, there it was! Just as predicted in my book, the appropriate change of the S-T segment smiled at me from the EKG's strip of paper. Fantastic! I leveled his dose at that point and he was successfully treated.

I had been so intent on the mechanics of this problem that I had overlooked the most basic indication of therapeutic success—he was breathing more easily and clearly felt better as his appetite, energy and complaints affirmed. Still, it was a good feeling, even though it had been cookbook therapy and the drug did all the work. I persuaded myself that I had something to do with it.

Late that afternoon I was reviewing the EKG and savoring this minor triumph when the nurse asked me to check on Joe. His breathing had become quite labored and he was now "asleep". In fact Joe was cyanotic and in coma. His blood pressure was unobtainable, his pulse very weak and he was sweating profusely. I applied the oxygen mask to his face and told the nurse to get some epinephrine and an endotracheal tube to insert into his main breathing tube.

While she was scrambling for the supplies I watched old Joe slip into death. He let out a deep breath, turned his face and died. All I could do was to let this inevitable transition occur right before my eyes, without altering it one micron. The mask continued to hiss oxygen and I let it persist, probably as a subconscious effort to will him alive again. I was humbled and subdued by my sense of helplessness.

Joan came to say goodbye to her father. She accepted his death with sadness and composure. The gurney carried Joe to the isolated little room in the basement of the hospital to await the arrival of the hearse from Gander, his burial site.

Five minutes later, the nurse had cleaned up the room with the efficiency that came from practice. I stared at the clean white sheets stretched tightly across the recently occupied bed for a while until I left to check on my living, breathing patients.

I fell asleep after supper and woke at 10 o'clock. It was black outside. Somewhere in that darkness a car was rushing along to beat the last midnight ferry run across the main tickle. I went out for a walk. My mind wandered, seeking escape from the tangible environment. I thought of Carol and Lynn back home and wondered what they were doing at this very moment. As a result of this, my first experience with death, life drew sharply into focus and I wished I were home in the comfort of my family.

It had been over a week since I had received a letter from Carol detailing Lynn's progress with reading. She wrote about our daughter, and not much about herself. At the time, I didn't think much of it, as all I wrote about were my discoveries in the actual practice of medicine, an opportunity beyond value for a fourth year medical student. Because she had quiet confidence in my abilities, apparently Carol saw nothing unusual in my care and treatment of patients so early in my medical career. It was enough that I knew of the extraordinary nature of this fellowship. In spite of the guilt I felt in the lengthy separation, I rationalized it with the benefit my experience will provide my patients in the future.

That night, the sky was ablaze with stars all glittering in different colors and sizes, arranged in every geometric form conceivable. Directly above me seemed the greatest concentration of stars imaginable, drifting off into extinction as my eye descended to the horizon. By hanging my head back and staring into the depths of a single point in the sky I was able to visualize more and more stars deeply distant and previously invisible.

Man can experience only what his physiology will allow, and what incredible things, what precious things must go entirely unnoticed because of our limited capacities. Our ears are constructed to hear sound of only certain frequencies, our eyes to see colors of only specific wavelengths. What procession of events was happening in that sky over my head, and yet invisible to me?

The moon captured my attention from these drifting thoughts. Its naked, tipped crescent seemed to hang in imbalance, weighted down by its shadowed sphere. The darkened circle had a soft, velvet, finely granular texture like that of an insects' compound eye when viewed beneath a microscope; and was the color of Russian caviar lightened by that faint suggestion of gray so exquisitely produced in a Steuben glass display.

Yet for all the glory and sparkle of these celestial carbon concentrations, they were unaware of their own existence. Only I had the capacity to say, "I think, therefore I am", to verify and recognize my own, and therefore their, existence. What a unique circumstance—for something to be capable of existence, and yet remain totally unaware of that state. As limited as I knew man to be, at that moment I felt we held a preferred status in the impersonal laws of physics and biology that govern our universe.

I stumbled, dizzy in thought. The distant glimmer of headlights bouncing off an invisible road in the darkness sobered me and returned me to the present. It was the people from Gander. Even though they had made this trip before, I directed the hearse behind the hospital where they backed up to the ground level windows.

We went into the basement. Joan stood near the gurney holding her father's body. Her arms hugging each other tightly, she leaned with her hip pressed against the gurney. At our appearance, she seemed to startle into awareness as she stepped away from the gurney. The mortician's team covered Joe with a blanket before straining to lift his heavy weight up onto the stretcher, then sliding him into the hearse.

To this day, I remember so clearly standing in that basement room looking out the window at the gleaming back panel of the hearse and the bright red taillights. The dark night summer sky framed the vehicle as heavy doors slammed behind the team. The deep throated muffler came to life. The taillights dimmed as the driver released his foot from the brake and pulled away. I watched the taillights disappear, swallowed by the night....the moonlight and the stars too far away to illuminate the road. This celestial imagery was made more vivid by the contrast of Joe's death.

At that time, I didn't feel responsible for his death. It was his two pack a day habit, his genetics, his age and absence of good health practice, so I'm not sure that his life could have been prolonged in a more modern hospital, with more extreme measures. Even so, I felt a deep sense of limitation. Being incapable of controlling life, powerless to prevent or postpone death, what was I doing in medicine? It would take me awhile to incorporate the fact that many conditions are not curable, giving me a broader perspective of the doctor's function.

CHAPTER SIXTEEN

THE BIRD ON THE LAWN

*"No one is thinking if everyone
is thinking alike."*
General George S. Patton

"Little Bitty Pretty One",
Clyde McPhatter, 1962

New problems consumed my attention.

The baby, Mary, had continued to vomit and now weighed less than 7 pounds. Her healthy pink faded into an unhealthy beige. The mosaic of blue veins visible as a subtle pattern beneath the infant's skin appeared dark and sluggish on Mary's dehydrated thigh. Pyloric stenosis became a greater possibility, so we attempted a fluoroscopy by feeding her barium with her milk. Like trying to input oral worming medicine into a piglet, it took two men and a nurse to hold her down long enough to get some barium laced milk into her system. Squirming and screaming, she wiggled and twisted, then promptly vomited out the mixture as soon as we released her.

"Colic," said the Old Man shaking his head and backing away from the crib. His tone was not as forceful as it had been, so I continued to gently press my case for pyloric stenosis.

Afternoon clinic also had its fill of challenges.

The inhabitants of Twillingate viewed medical help as a last resort. After grandma's mustard and herb panaceas failed for the third time, the secret family tea remedy resulted in more rather than less vomiting, and nailing garlic to the door jamb did not reduce the swelling in the abdomen, the ailing person would reluctantly drag himself into the clinic. While waiting for their appointment, they would glance at the door as if awaiting the appearance of a savior to alleviate their symptoms before having to actually be treated by the doctor. This 16th century concept of medical attention—something to be avoided when possible, and to be feared when inevitable—-often prevented a disorder from being treated when it was still manageable or curable.

Many patients presented with diseases in rather advanced stages when the diagnosis was fairly obvious. In fact, it was usually obvious even to the patient who otherwise would not have sought help. Such was the case of a 38 year-old man who I heard coughing in the waiting room for 20 minutes before I had a chance to see him. Thin, bug eyed, with sunken cheeks, he was weak, pale and looked sick. As unscientific as "looking sick" seems, it is really a very important observation to make about a patient. His face or skin color may be a subtle indication of a disease process somewhere in his body, and there is no question that cancer may manifest itself in this insidious way.

On examination he was indeed sick. His chest contained an area of abnormally increased breath sounds just over the right scapula, and a chest x-ray revealed an area of consolidation in the right upper lung field. My primary diagnosis was active tuberculosis, so I admitted him to a private room with isolation precautions.

This categorization meant he wore a mask at all times, and anyone entering the room wore a mask. The term "precautions" applies to the patient with a communicable illness, so visitors must wear masks and gowns for their own protection; "reverse precautions" means that the patient has so few bacteria fighting defenses of his own, as in advanced leukemia, that he himself must be protected against the normal bacteria from exposure to his visitors. He, as well as all visitors, must wear a mask to supplement his reduced natural defenses against infection. Another example of a patient who requires reverse precautions is one who has received a transplanted organ such as heart or kidney, and is on powerful drugs that suppress his natural ability to reject the donated organ. The disadvantage of such drugs is that they also suppress the ability to reject, or defend against, other foreign bodies, such as bacteria, and therefore infections, especially pneumonia, are a constant threat.

I performed a TB test by injecting a very small amount of fluid into the skin of his forearm. This fluid contained particles of protein from the cell wall of the bacteria that emulate TB (one cannot contract TB from this test). If the body has been infected by TB it will have produced TB fighting antibodies which bind to the TB protein, producing a large red swelling on the arm at the site of injection. This reaction is exactly what happened, and arrangements were made to fly him out by seaplane as soon as possible. Now that the diagnosis had been made, no one wanted any contact with him at all.

The seaplane was scheduled to arrive that afternoon, and someone had to take him out by boat. Mike and I drew lots—he lost. Although generally bully-bully, Mike was really uptight about this guy, even though I had been taking care of him. He tried to protest, but a bet was a bet. So with great reluctance he helped the patient down the short road from the hospital to the harbor. They both wore bright green surgical masks. It was a funny scene, the two of them in their masks facing each other with Mike rowing the boat to the seaplane and the patient sitting in the stern holding his small suitcase in his lap. After the patient had been helped on to the seaplane, Mike rowed back to the dock, still wearing his mask. In spite of his fears, we both survived the exposure to TB.

A few days later, a man in his mid-fifties with a full beard and Andy Rooney eyebrows walked in holding one hand with the other. The index finger on his left hand looked more like a Bratwurst than a digit as it pointed at me in the examination room. After introducing himself, he reported a month of progressive swelling from the knuckle to his fingertip, now nearly twice normal size. It looked like an infection, but he had no pain or redness, two hallmarks of an acute bacterial infection. Also there was no evidence of pus so there was nothing to drain. There was no history of a fishhook puncture wound or other trauma. I concluded he had sustained a trivial injury that had gone unnoticed at the time, and had now progressed to a significant problem. I gave him antibiotics.

He returned a week later with no improvement, so I turned to my encyclopedia of information—the Old Man. He chuckled and explained that this was a fairly common phenomenon in Twillingate known as "seal finger". Men walk out on the frozen bay in winter to slaughter an occasional stray seal. They grab the seal with their left hand and use a knife for the kill. Evidently, the seal carries a fungal parasite that penetrates the skin of the index or middle finger of the Newfie foolish enough not to wear a glove—a fitting revenge from the seal's point of view.

"Antibiotics won't do a damn bit of good, Richard. Just leave it alone and the finger will fall off on its own". The Old Man turned and left me standing there with my mouth open… at his unconcern about the fisherman losing a finger, and second, at my own feelings of stupidity for not determining the source of the swelling. Who knew?

We had never covered "seal finger" in med school! What I didn't know was the process of seal finger eventually led to a condition known as "dry gangrene" in which the finger slowly, progressively shrank down and atrophied into a black, hard petrified nubbin. The parasite continues to enjoy its success over the host organism, at least on a local level. As the parasite and its secondary inflammatory process continue to advance on the vascular supply to the digit, the index finger finds its blood supply cut off, essentially representing suicide on the part of the parasite that dies along with the dead finger. Eventually, the finger fell off on its own, leaving a remnant stump near the knuckle.

This is in stark contrast to the feared "wet gangrene". Here infection resides insidiously deep in the tissues, grows and foments in the rich nutrients provided by the surrounding tissue which may be deprived of blood inflow (arterial supply), but still has blood flow returning to the heart (venous drainage). The infection, in the absence of antibiotics and surgical attention, will gnaw its way further and further up the extremity like a brush fire gone wild, turn the entire arm (or leg) into a putrefying swamp of purulent necrotic tissue, enter the bloodstream and disseminate to the far corners of the body, implanting its bacterial brethren into the brain, heart, liver, bone marrow, joints and kidneys. This devastating assault is unrelenting, and leads to ferocious sepsis, multiple organ failure and, prior to modern medicine, the final event that blessedly removes all pain and fear: unconsciousness, cardio-pulmonary collapse and death.

Late one afternoon as things were winding down in the clinic, a distraught woman came in cradling a towel in her arms and pleading for immediate attention. There in the towel was her cat, indeed a rather sickly and somnolent cat who she claimed had been shot by a pellet gun wielded by a mischievous neighbor boy.

One problem—neither Mike nor I were veterinarians. Nor was I a surgeon or Mike a veterinary anesthesiologist...but we were about to impersonate both.

None of the three "real" doctors were available for advice and, of course, there was no vet on the island, so we took cat into the x-ray room for an x-ray. Aha! Just as we suspected! The cat had been shot by a pellet gun and there on the x-ray film, floating somewhere around the cat's abdomen was a pellet. After a brief discussion we concluded surgery was necessary.

Like Laurel and Hardy, we went to the waiting room and presented the x-ray to the woman. She reluctantly agreed with our plan, which really was the only chance the cat had—a poor chance at that. We closed the clinic door behind us and Mike proceeded to anesthetize the cat while I arranged the necessary surgical instruments. The cat seemed to vigorously disagree with our plan as Mike placed a few drops of chloroform on a sponge and gently placed it over the cat's nose. With that the cat emerged from its somnolent state and scratched the shit out of Mike's hand. Undeterred, Mike rolled the cat in a towel and repeated the process, this time with more than just a few drops of chloroform. The cat promptly expired.

"Jesus, Mike! You OD'd the cat on chloroform!"

"Dick, quick, open the cat up and get the damn pellet out! We can't tell the lady this was an anesthetic death!"

"Why not?"

Mike wanted to shift the blame from his incompetence to mine, from an anesthetic death to a surgical death. It seemed the lesser of two evils and I agreed. I made a quick midline incision in the now dead cat's belly, extracted the pellet and dropped it in a metal pan with an audible "plunk" for all to hear on the far side of the clinic door. After an appropriate moment of delay, Drs. Laurel and Hardy shuffled into the waiting room with the pan and pellet in hand. Needless to say, the woman's reaction was not what we hoped for—she saw right through our white lab coats to the very incompetents that we were. I felt badly for the cat, badly for the woman and badly for us. 0 for 3.

CHAPTER SEVENTEEN

BAPTISM

"Sometimes, getting an education is like getting a sip of water out of a fire hose."
Thomas B. Humphreys, Sr. (Cdr. USN Ret.)

"Doubt whom you will, but never yourself."
Christian Nestell Bovee

Newfies have a very distinct dialect all their own, and though basically English, it is very difficult to understand. It took me three weeks before I picked up the verbal short-cuts and slang words, and even then I was fooled often.

One afternoon, a mother entered the clinic trailed by her five children like steps on the stairs from the oldest girl, about age twelve, to a four-year old boy. When I asked what the problem was, she pointed to the little boy and said, "Es ave a fection in ees ire."

"An infection in his hair?" I replied. Scabies was very common there and I thought this is what he had. So I looked carefully all over his head for about five minutes, separating the hair and shining my light on his scalp in search of the tell tale red evidence.

Nothing. Absolutely nothing.

Trying to maintain a degree of professional cool, I turned to her and said, "An infection where?"

She grabbed his right ear and repeated, "In ees ire, in ees ire". Yes indeed, he surely did. A rip roaring otitis media with pus in the ear canal. I reassured the mother that his hair was all right and then gave her some penicillin for her son's ear infection. I felt like a jerk!

Ward rounds often produced a few surprises as well. Rounds were made on all patients every day at 5 in the afternoon. I was used to the starch and formality of rounds done in crisp hospital whites. We walked behind the professor in order of rank, i.e. Chief Resident, Junior Resident, slave (short for intern), stud (short for 4th year student) and gnome (short for 3rd year student).

However, here in Twillingate, professional attire was casual, to say the least. The Old Man always wore a pair of worn out gray chino pants and an open shirt. The only instrument he ever carried was an old Navy surplus flashlight, which he used more as a night stick than to illuminate anything. Instead of starched whites and a respectful distance in the rear, I followed our fearless leader with my stethoscope stuck in my dungaree pocket.

Despite the informality, the Old Man commanded our complete respect on rounds, and he determined the pace. He stopped at every bed, at least to say hello if nothing more. One woman, by reputation a chronic complainer, was prepared with a new problem as the Old Man approached her bed. Morbidly obese didn't begin to describe her size. Her hair a frizzy henna red in a halo of curls around her circular face gave her the appearance of a pumpkin atop a sand pile. "I hurts all over," was her greeting to Dr. John. Followed by, "I can't gets out of bed."

With a frown, he strolled to her bedside and pulled down the covers. Gently grabbing a huge roll of her abdomen, he said, "If I had this, I'd have a hard time getting out of bed, too". The woman nodded in silent agreement, viewing the expanse of her exposed abdomen.

This exchange was quite typical of his doctor-patient relationships. In many respects, the patients considered themselves his children so they expected verbal discipline from him. Dr. John expressed subdued displeasure when he mumbled under his breath. He had a sixth sense about his "children" and did not tolerate any frivolous or devious complaints. They understood this and took a degree of comfort in it, and tested him occasionally just to see that his paternal attitude was still there. He was greatly admired, more than anyone in the community.

The next patient, a 23 year-old female who looked much younger, stared out her window and answered his questions in a monotone. She didn't face him, apparently preferring the trees and sky to her doctor. Something about her demeanor interested me so I made a note of her name, Jane Beridge. Mousy brown hair pulled tightly into a pony tail resulted in her thin face appearing gaunt. Without a line on her face, she looked like a high school student.

Recently a neurology specialist had diagnosed her with petit mal epilepsy, characterized by short spells of blank staring and inattention to the environment, without loss of consciousness. She was taking Dilantin twice a day as prescribed by the specialist, but there didn't seem to be any improvement. I thought back to the psychiatry unit, and remembered patients with petit mal were started on Tridione. Only grand mal epileptics were given Dilantin.

After rounds, I returned the books and to read up on it again. Cecil & Loeb (the internal medicine bible) did not mention Dilantin as therapy for petit mal epilepsy. Jane was Al's patient, so I spoke to him about my findings. It never occurred to him to challenge the treatment since it had been prescribed by a "specialist". However, he was willing to give her a trial of Tridione, and discontinued Dilantin immediately. Knowing it would take several days for the Tridione to work, I switched her medication that day.

Most doctors have built up a veneer of pride and ego that would result in a protective response when their clinical judgment is challenged. Not Al. He was so low key, or perhaps it was just a lack of professional interest, that he quietly and without resistance acquiesced to my intervention on behalf of his patient. Never have I encountered another physician that would match the subdued ego of Al. (Or perhaps it was an open mind, unusual in physicians in those days.)

Sitting two beds away from Jane was a very pretty 17 year-old girl named Kathleen. Kathleen was unique, not only because she was pretty but because her face was always scrubbed clean and her hair neatly combed. She sat Indian style on her bed awaiting our rounds. As a rule, personal appearance was of little interest to these Newfies, and personal hygiene seemed irrelevant. Very few people used toothbrushes, and with the influx of civilization in the form of candy bars, licorice and chewing gum, most people were totally edentulous (toothless) by age 30. Many teenagers had lost all of their front teeth, a pathetic spectacle since prosthetic devices were unavailable (much like the dental woes of the people in Appalachia today).

By contrast, Kathleen had a full set of beautiful teeth, and her whole presence was rather incongruous because she looked so alert and healthy. She was not my patient, but my curiosity piqued when I saw her on rounds day after day for over a week.

When I finished ordering the Tridione for Jane at the nurse's station, I picked up Kathleen's chart. "Patient complains of pain in her right mid-back. URI (upper respiratory infection) with associated cough for one week. Chest suspicious. Admit for possible pneumonia". That had been written by Al one week earlier when she had been admitted to the hospital. No antibiotics had been ordered, and no subsequent note written other than "Chest clear" recorded four days ago. Her low grade fever persisted. Since she wasn't my patient, I didn't want to presume, but it did seem that a more adequate evaluation was indicated. I returned to her bedside and asked her a few questions.

"How do you feel today, Kathleen?"

"I finds it in ma side – ere". She placed the palm of her right hand over her kidney area on the right side of her back. A patient with pneumonia can have pain in this area, but it is usually well localized and they will point to the area with one or two fingers to emphasize its localized nature. She used her entire hand, as an indication that the pain was more diffuse and possibly originated from the kidney instead of the lung.

"Does it hurt when you take in a deep breath?" Pneumonia will spread to involve the delicate membranous lining of the inside of the chest wall, and this will produce localized pain on deep inspiration.

"No sir".

"Does it burn when you pass your urine?"

"Yes sir. It burns".

That just about clinched the diagnosis for UTI (urinary tract infection). I listened to her lungs which were entirely clear. I gently tapped over the area of her kidney and she winced slightly. This valuable sign is known as CVA (costo-vertebral angle) pain, and always directs attention to the kidneys. Microscopic examination of her urine showed many red and white cells and many bacteria. I jotted a note on her chart. "Patient now complains of dysuria, chills and fever. Exam reveals clear chest, right CVA tenderness. Urine analysis – many RBC's and WBC's/HPF, loaded with motile bacteria. Impression – UTI. Rx – Gantrisin, 3 gm po stat, then 1 gm/po/qid".

It was no great triumph on my part to make this diagnosis. As a matter of fact, I criticized myself for not having been more observant and suspicious earlier. And the diagnosis was rather obvious. Al had not bothered to do even a rudimentary evaluation, and had failed to follow her daily clinical course. I said nothing, but lost respect for him because of such medical laxity. He had violated a basic lesson of medicine that I remembered from earlier training—you can make a wrong diagnosis from the right facts, and that may be a forgivable mistake. But you can never make a correct diagnosis from wrong or grossly inadequate facts, and that is not forgivable. This is a truism in medicine that applies to knowledgeable specialists as well as med students (it is characteristic of the quack to disregard facts, since he does not know how to interpret them). I did not have the experience or confidence to make the right diagnosis in many cases, so by way of compensation I naturally intensified my efforts to get an accurate history and perform a careful exam.

The next morning the Old Man operated on the now 6 pound 5 oz. baby and corrected her pyloric stenosis. My impression was vindicated, but the Old Man was reserved in his acknowledgement of my diagnostic coup (translation: one's greatest satisfaction comes from within, not from grasping for false praise from others). The wall of the stomach and canal which leads into the duodenum had a greatly enlarged muscle layer, so enlarged that it was obstructing the canal itself. So the Old Man took the scalpel and made a longitudinal incision along this canal through the outer covering and through the thick muscle wall down to the inner most layer, the stomach lining (or mucosa) where he stopped. This simple procedure, called a pyloromyotomy or Ramstead procedure, completely relieved the obstruction and cured the child of her problem. Rapid cure is one of the rewarding aspects of surgery. It offers very direct gratification, and the surgeon's involvement is aggressive and straightforward.

As the case was finishing up, a nurse popped in and told me one of the Mounties was downstairs and he wanted to see Mike and me. Immediately pangs of guilt replaced my feelings of satisfaction at the conclusion of the successful surgery. I racked my brain to think of something we might have done to have upset the local constabulary. So Mike and I held a brief discussion before going downstairs.

Two un-mounted Canadian Mounties served as the local police force for the island. They had a small headquarters near the fishery supplied with short wave radio gear, and an imposing yellow Buick with a big black shield-like emblem on the doors advertising them as the Royal Police. Very little ever occurred that demanded their presence, but it was comforting to have them as insurance. Except for one thing. The inhabitants were definitely restricted in alcohol consumption by Canadian law, as is still the case throughout Canada. It was more than a minor infraction to be caught with an oversupply. There were two local bars, but the seemingly ubiquitous Mounties provided enough anxiety that serious drinking was an underground accomplishment.

We were not guilty in this respect, and the only thing we could come up with was a small beach party we had held with some of the hospital personnel a few nights before. It had been a great party, and had turned into an unexpected fish feast. Small, sardine-sized jet black fish, capelin, swarm the shores of Newfoundland in mid-July to spawn. The females lay their eggs in shallow water and the males deposit sperm to fertilize the eggs. For an unknown reason most of them die after this week long process. During spawning the capelin choke the shore waters in a ten or twelve foot wide band, literally millions of them churning the water in all directions. This phenomenon occurs all over Newfoundland, so the number of capelin spawning must be astronomic.

We brought a large pot and a bunch of paper plates, and built a fire on the beach from driftwood. Mike waded into the icy water. Although it was July, the water was frigid, and huge icebergs floated by all summer as close as three to four miles from shore. He dipped the pot in and came up with a load of squirming capelin. We put the pot on the fire and ate boiled capelin to our hearts content. All this occurred at 11 o'clock at night and I figured our laughter had disturbed a few of the locals.

I figured wrong.

We had neglected to extinguish the fire completely, and a few smoldering embers remained the next morning.

The constable gave us mild admonishment which I thought was fair enough, and that was that. But it was not good to have them on our bad side, so we decided to be a bit more conservative during our off hours.

As luck would have it, we messed up again several weeks later. The hospital owned a VW van micro bus which functioned as a grocery truck, ambulance, weekend tour car and anything else we could think of to get away from the hospital from time to time. I think Mike's secret ambition was to compete at Le Mans, for he horsed that VW around as fast as he could, especially outside the village where the chances of getting caught were slim. He failed to exhibit any discretion in town either, so it was only a matter of time before something happened.

One afternoon late in July, we had gone to the store for some bogus purpose, and on the return trip Mike sped over a rock which flew up and hit a pedestrian in the leg. Fortunately, it was no more than a bruise, but we didn't know it had happened so we continued on our way back to the hospital. The next day we received our second visit from the constable, who, since he didn't know which of us had been driving, threatened to confiscate both our licenses. He was nice enough about the whole thing, but reasonably disturbed and wasn't about to put up with much more. Mike decided it was time to tread lightly, and tried to mend his lead footed ways for the rest of the summer.

Mike was really an interesting fellow. He was broad minded and very rational about most things, but ridiculously narrow-minded and persistent about others—such as driving fast and the importance of British titles. He would always sign his name "Esq." and added on several graduate titles the following year when he became a doctor. In addressing letters to him after he returned to London I would purposely delete the string of abbreviated titles that followed his name, and this peeved him to no end. As roommates we got along well and had very few incompatibilities. And he taught me the words to "Rule Britannia".

We agreed from the beginning of the summer that we would alternate on call duty at night. Our room was in a small wing added onto the side of the hospital which had the advantage of allowing us to take duty from our room, so we often had a full night's sleep. However, this arrangement had the disadvantage of waking both of us up when the nurse would summon whoever was on duty by a non-discriminating fist on the door. There was no way to avoid this since anything less than pounding failed to wake either of us.

One memorable night, after Mike had had his fill of delivering babies in the middle of the night, he told the nurses that they could do the night deliveries themselves. They were trained to do this, but if any complications arose they were to call him. I had only spent four weeks in Ob-Gyn during my third year, and I was just as glad to have Mike handle obstetrical complications with which I had little experience. Frantic pounding jerked us awake.

"Delivery!" the nurse's voice through the door.

So I closed my ears and rolled over. Mike had obviously done the same thing for the pounding persisted. He finally got up and stumbled to the door, mumbled something to the nurse, then flicked on the overhead light.

"What's the matter, Mike?" I mumbled. "And can you turn out the light?"

"Nurse thinks it's a breach and I've got to see to get dressed. Sorry".

Silence for a moment before I heard him sit on his bed. "Christ, Dick, do you realize it's quarter of four? I'll be damned if I'm going to get dressed to deliver a baby at quarter of four in the morning." So he pulled on his very British crimson dressing gown, complete with black satin lapels, jammed his feet into a pair of loafers and clomped off down the corridor.

This was something I couldn't miss, so camera and flashbulb in hand I followed him to the OR. It was quite a scene. The woman lay on her back on the table with her legs up and open for delivery. Covered with green drapes, her head thrashed from side to side but otherwise she was pretty stoical. Two large pans were on the floor serving only to get in the way as far as I could see. One nurse was taking the patient's blood pressure while the other was adjusting the overhead lights. A pair of forceps lay on the Mayo stand with sterile sponges, instruments and suture material.

Her ruptured membranes had dumped water on the floor surrounding the table. The lighting, the commotion, the mess on the floor contributed to the atmosphere of a World War I first-aid station. In the midst of this stood Mike, crimson dressing gown, rolled up sleeves, sterile gloves and surgical mask. All in living color which I captured in a snapshot. This was a far cry from the organized, controlled setting of the deliveries at the University hospital. Mike delivered a baby boy who promptly peed all over his arms. The crimson dressing gown somehow escaped damage.

CHAPTER EIGHTEEN

SEAT OF MY PANTS

*"A discovery is an accident meeting a
prepared mind."*
Albert Szent-Gyorgyi, biochemist

"Moments to Remember",
The Four Lads, 1955

I had my eventful nights as well. In addition to being
on duty for the hospital we were simultaneously on call for
the whole village. One of the few bona fide times that I had
to use the VW came late one night in response to a call from
Darrell's Arm, a remote part of the island that jutted out from
the surrounding land. A family had sent their 14 year-old son
on his bicycle to the hospital to summon a doctor. I threw on
my clothes, grabbed my stethoscope and bag and headed for
the VW. Not expecting any intelligible description of the
problem, I somewhat casually asked the boy what the trouble
was as we climbed into the van.

"My grandpa can't breathe well." That was a good
enough description for what could be an asthmatic attack or
heart failure among many other possibilities. That was about
the extent of the history he could give me so I ran back inside
to grab an ampule of morphine sulfate and one of epinephrine, a syringe and a couple of alcohol packets. We jumped
in the VW van and drove over the bumpy, potholed, stone-
flying dirt road in the dark of a Newfoundland night. Pitch

black. Seven minutes later we arrived at the boy's home, a weather beaten, bent over shack of a place with the dull light of an oil lamp shining from a window like a one-eyed old man.

He wasn't kidding either. His grandfather, about 80 years old, was lying down in bed propped up to one side by two pillows so that he rested partially on his left elbow. He was taking rapid and deep breaths at the rate of nearly 30 a minute, tightening his neck muscles and extending his head back with every inspiration to facilitate his efforts. He neck veins bulged out during exhalation and there was an audible rattle in his throat as if he were breathing through a film of water. The lighting from an oil lamp was lousy at best, and every time I leaned in to examine him, he disappeared in my shadow.

We carried him to the main room and sat him on the couch. His pulse was 120, rapid and weak, his skin wet and clammy. I listened to his chest which was filled with wet, crackly sounds called rales, indicative of fluid in the tiny air pockets of the lungs. His pajamas were soaked with urine, giving off the distinctive odor of nitrogen compounds.

This was a classic case of severe congestive heart failure, or pulmonary edema. Fluid was backing up in his lungs because of a failing heart, and he was drowning in it. I knew the diagnosis, but now what?

Keeping my stethoscope against his chest as a stalling tactic, as if I knew what I was doing, I summoned the methods of treating pulmonary edema from my panicky mind.

My pulse was over 100, rapid and strong.

I had a stone silent audience.

I recalled a mnemonic that we had learned in med school—MOST are DAMP and used this as a guideline. God! What if they knew I was treating their grandfather from a memorized mnemonic?! Well it was all I had and at that point I needed all the help I could get. Let's see—morphine, oxygen, sit up, tourniquets.

First things first.

I broke open the ampoule of morphine and drew up all 10 mgm. That seemed too much, so I injected 5 mgm directly into his arm vein over a minute's time, trying to keep the needle from penetrating through the vein wall as the grandfather puffed and moved about. I withdrew the needle and took care to save the remaining morphine, now dark red from the blood I had drawn back into the syringe before the injection.

He was developing a large hematoma in his arm where the needle had left a hole in the vein, so I had his daughter hold the alcohol sponge tightly against the swelling while at the same time she helped to keep him upright. This eased his breathing a little, giving me a moment to think.

What am I going to do for oxygen?

Punt.

No oxygen in the van, so forget that.

What's next? Tourniquets. The theory, and it works, is to apply loose tourniquets around the arms and legs, no more than three at a time, so as to reduce blood flow back to the already overloaded heart and lungs, and yet still allow arterial blood to be pumped into the limbs. In essence, fluid is transferred to the arms and legs and reduced in the lungs.

I had no tourniquets with me but they were easy enough to make with a towel and a couple of belts. I applied them to both thighs and left biceps area, testing the pulse beyond the tourniquet to make sure that I had not cut off the arterial blood supply.

That took care of MOST.

The stone-silent family looked at me as if they assumed I knew what I was doing. Or so I hoped. Now for DAMP. Digitalis to strengthen the heartbeat—none with me; aminophylline to dilate the bronchial tubes by relaxing the muscles in their walls—also none; Damn! mercuhydrin, a diuretic—none, and I don't know the dose anyhow; phlebotomy, or drawing off blood to reduce blood volume and lessen the strain on the heart. That was a little risky so I thought I would hold off for awhile.

Since the urgency of the situation had eased off a little, I became more aware of the family in the room. It was a very modest house with warped wood floors covered by a few faded scattered rugs. The furniture was mostly handmade, except for the couch which was a relic from somewhere in the attic. A very plain picture of Jesus Christ hung on the wall nearest the door. There were no magazines or books, no radio or television. The room was dimly lit from two oil lamps. Grandmother sat very quietly in a deep upholstered chair, almost swallowed up in its frame, hands in lap and staring continuously at one spot on the floor. Her expression was not one of grief, fear or anxiety, but reflected a deep weariness and perhaps resignation.

It seemed so strange, these two who had the most in common seemed really to have the least in common, a certain detachment. The father stood behind me, his son dozing under his left arm and a belt dangling from his right hand. Like a dutiful scrub nurse waiting patiently to hand an instrument to the surgeon, the son held his belt. His faith in my authority was in stark contrast to my own lack of confidence. His wife remained seated next to her father on the couch, supporting his arm and toweling his forehead and face.

Large blue rheumy eyes darted around the room as the patient seemed suspicious of this temporary reprieve, daring not to do anything to upset a delicate balance, which for the moment seemed to be in his favor. He presented a strangely asymmetric appearance with belts placed unequally on either thigh gathering the material of his pajama legs, and a bulky half-tied towel around his arm.

Trying to look functional, I periodically checked his pulse and listened to his chest. No one said anything. They didn't offer help and they asked no questions. But he did seem to be improving slightly. His pulse was down to 100, his respirations less deep. I guess my optimism was shared by the family for the daughter offered me some tea and cod. Of course I couldn't say no. This involved feeding the black, iron wood-burning stove with sticks of kindling until adequate heat developed. She produced two pieces of salted cod from a small bin and placed them in a frying pan. A pot of tea which had been sitting beside the stove was reheated over the flat skillet next to the cod. These were new sensations to me, new odors and I enjoyed the opportunity to briefly divert my attention from grandfather. I felt humbled by the efforts needed to provide this meal for me in the middle of the night. She was showing appreciation infinitely more sincerely (and more gratifying to me) than a completed Blue Cross/Blue Shield insurance form.

I ate the cod which tasted like a salt lick, trying inconspicuously to dilute it with the unsweetened tea. It was a difficult chore to get it all down and even manage a smile. The husband helped me carry grandfather into the VW and supported him as I drove back to the hospital. We put him in the nearest available room but the stress of transportation had made his breathing somewhat worse. I had a long night ahead of me so I didn't protest when the husband said he would walk back on his own, in the dark nonetheless.

I asked the nurse to get grandfather some oxygen. The next step was a base-line EKG and a slow IV drip. There was no evidence of a heart attack. I gave him digitalis IV, and placed 500 mgm of aminophyllin in the IV bottle. It was now 5 o'clock in the morning and I was certain he was doing better than I was at this point. So I wrote his orders in the chart and handed them to the nurse to read before I left:

1. Bed rest
2. Vital signs – blood pressure, pulse, temperature q4h
3. NPO (nothing by mouth)
4. To be supported in sitting position no less than 60 degrees at all times (this is to impede the venous blood flow from his legs back to the heart in order to lessen the strain on the struggling right ventricle, and to ease his respiration at the same time)
5. Oxygen by mask—5 liters/minute
6. IV fluid—1 liter D5W with 500 mgm aminophylin to run at 50 cc/hour
7. Digoxin .125 mgm IV stat (given)
8. Complete I & O (record all fluids given and all fluids put out by the patient, e.g. urine)

9.   Urinal at bedside—measure and record

10. Call me stat for complications

Fortunately, there were no complications that night and I returned to my bed for 2 ½ hours of beautiful, undisturbed sleep.

Back at his bedside at 7:40 A.M., I checked his vitals. He looked extremely weak from the prolonged efforts of fighting for air, but his pulse was 98 and his respiration was much quieter. His temperature was 99.6, a sign of possible infection starting in his lungs. I tracked this closely. His chest still contained a few rales at both lung bases, but was much improved over his prior status. His urine output was quite adequate, an encouraging sign. I ordered a chest x-ray and an EKG, reassured him that he was doing better and left for the OR.

The first case was a hernia repair in a young man who had developed a bulge in his right groin two weeks earlier, after lifting heavy crates at the fishery. Examination indicated an inguinal hernia and surgical repair had been scheduled that morning.

We decided to do the repair under spinal anesthesia. In principal this makes more sense than a general anesthetic. Why put the entire patient asleep when all you need is half his body asleep? Furthermore, general anesthesia involves greater risks than spinal anesthesia, though such risks have been minimized in the current era. Potential problems with general anesthesia include a sudden drop in blood pressure, vomiting into the anesthesia mask and heart irregularities. These demand constant attention during a general. Also, the patient is usually unable to eat until the day following surgery and post-operative pneumonia is more common.

In contrast, recovering from a spinal simply involves lying in bed waiting for the Novocaine to wear off so you can move your legs again. The spinal patient is allowed meals following surgery and the incidence of pneumonia is very low.

The patient lay on the operating table. I spent a minute explaining what I was going to do before placing him on his left side.

"Curl up in a ball," I said. This position draws the tapered end of the spinal cord above the level of the small of the back, so a long spinal needle can be safely inserted where it will penetrate only the dura and spinal fluid without injuring the cord itself.

I washed the small of his back with a sponge soaked in iodine solution that caused a reddish discoloration, starting right over the spine and working outward in circles. Then I repeated this with alcohol, further sterilizing the skin and cleaning off the iodine at the same time. After draping the spinal area I felt for the space between two lumbar vertebral bones and injected a small amount of Novacaine into the skin. In another syringe I drew up 10 mgm of Pontocaine (a spinal anesthetic) and mixed it with an equal volume of heavy sugar solution. This made it denser and heavier than the watery spinal fluid and would prevent the Pontocaine from moving upward along the spinal cord and potentially paralyzing his muscles of respiration. Thus the Pontocaine would follow gravity and safely remain in the lower part of the spinal fluid to provide anesthesia for only the lower abdomen and legs.

I inserted the long spinal needle through the numbed skin and slowly down through muscle and fascia until I felt the characteristic pop of the dura giving way. Clear spinal fluid started to drip back out of the needle. Victory! I had struck pay dirt! Can you imagine if the patient knew how inexperienced I really was? I attached the prepared syringe and injected the Pontocaine solution. I removed the needle and placed the patient on his back with his legs tipped slightly down for the gravity effect on the Pontocaine. In a few minutes he felt his toes and legs going numb and I scrubbed up.

After telling the Old Man everything was ready, I stood quietly at the table with my hands resting on the sterile drapes which hid everything but a small area of his groin.

The Old Man, gowned and gloved, approached the other side of the table. Instead of saying anything, asking for anything, he simply stood there in silence.

After a slight delay he nodded to me.

My eyes widened as I realized this was it, the opportunity I thought would not happen for another two years. No time to let anxiety replace the calm confidence I had felt seconds ago—-when I was just going to assist. A deep breath…

"Knife, please" I said, my voice sounding like it was coming from someone else. And she handed me the knife.

As I was about to make the incision slightly lower than necessary, the Old Man gently guided my hand to the right place. I drew the knife in a small arc and began my first hernia operation. I was surprised how easily the blade descended through the dermis and into the subcutaneous fatty tissue. There was very little bleeding which was easily controlled by mild pressure from the small retractors placed on either side of the wound.

Here I was, in control of the knife, while the Old Man retracted for me—what a rush! There at the base of the incision was a glistening external oblique fascia whose fibers run in parallel and anchor onto the pubic bone. A small U-shaped opening in the fascia allows for the exit of the spermatic cord in the male (in the female, it is nothing but a rudimentary small fibrous band of little significance).

In the growing embryo, the gonads (ovaries and testes) both develop inside the lower abdomen. The ovaries forever remain in this position while the testes and supporting spermatic cord descend into the scrotum for a cooler environment as required for viable sperm (an un-descended testicle is often non-functional). During this descent, the testes leave a tract, a weak point through which bowel can follow and actually descend straight into the scrotum. If the bowel cannot be pushed back up, it is incarcerated (trapped). If swelling progresses and cuts off the bowel blood supply, it is strangulated and becomes a dire surgical emergency.

My patient had the simplest form wherein the patent tract was allowing an occasional knuckle of bowel to swell in the groin without troublesome descent into the scrotum.

I incised the fascia parallel to its fibers and identified the ileo-inguinal nerve which provides sensation to the skin over the groin. I easily pushed, or reduced, the knuckle of bowel back into the abdomen and over-sewed the defect with multiple interrupted sutures of 3-0 silk. I tied each suture very deliberately with two complete square knots (a square knot does not slip), taking great care to respect and avoid injury to the "NAVY triad", or femoral Nerve, Artery and Vein (NAV), lying and pulsating just below my index finger. Better to drive the suture into my own finger than into NAV, so during suture placement my index finger rested diligently over this dangerous anatomy.

As I held up the suture lines, the Old Man took the suture scissors and cut the silk ties at a 45 degree angle, just above the knot, a nice technical trick to avoid cutting the knot itself. I irrigated the wound with warm normal saline, closed the divided fascia with running 4-0 silk suture material, and approximated the skin with nylon suture. In experienced hands, 15 minutes skin to skin (incision to closure). In my tentative hands, with all the help I could ask for, 57 minutes skin to skin! At the end of the case, one word came from the Old Man—"Good". I think he was being generous.

CHAPTER NINETEEN

DAY IN THE LIFE

"Victories that are easy are cheap. Those only are worth having which come as a result of hard fighting."
Henry Ward Beecher, clergyman

"Send in the Clowns",
Judy Collins, 1975

It was a sunny but cool Sunday and the summer moved along. Mike and I took the van out for a spin, this time to the uninhabited northwestern edge of the island where the land rose to huge, jagged cliffs ending precipitously in the water 300 feet below. There was no beach and giant columns of rock, like fallen Greek ruins, lay in the deep clear waters. I side armed a smooth flat stone straight out. It paused and then fell in slow motion, creeping its way back to shore as it descended. It produced a barely perceptible scar in the water which was quickly healed and forgotten. Far below me hanging close to the cliff were several seagulls, discrete specks of white against the immense background of the dark green ocean. Each gull's motion cancelled out the others, so that they seemed to remain in a perpetual, but motionless circle.

We sat on the warm, dry grass airing our minds in silent appreciation for this respite from the hospital.

Then he started to laugh.

"I was just thinking of my first patient here," he chortled. "I mean my very first patient. It was that pig I fixed up."

I didn't know it had been his first patient but I did remember Pig. Pig had developed a prolapsed rectum and was sicker than stink from diarrhea. Mike was wandering around the hospital wards his first day when the nurse told him someone was in the clinic to be seen. It was the man who owned the pig, so Mike trudged up to his house, stethoscope in his back pocket and a rectal glove on. The only thing that facilitated examination and treatment was that pig was so exhausted he couldn't struggle well. So Mike requested a surgical consultation with the old man and the two of them worked out a plan of attack. They held the pig down on his side while making a small painless hole in the back wall of the prolapsed rectum. He then reinserted the rectum and placed a pack through the hole into the surrounding tissues. That was all there was to it, and two weeks later he removed the pack which by then had caused enough scar tissue and reaction to hold the rectum in place.

Pig was cured and as far as his owner was concerned Mike was the original Albert Schweitzer. He offered Mike his horse anytime he wanted to ride. The only trouble was the horse was a sway-back plow-puller type and the rocky, hilly terrain restricted the "ride" to a slow walk. Mike collected his first fee and went for a ride that afternoon.

We told patient stories for a while and had some good laughs. One was about a girl I saw in clinic who had gotten a fishhook caught deep in the pad of her thumb. We had not covered that subject in medical school and I struggled with that damn thing for about 20 minutes, persuading, cajoling, manipulating, all to no avail. I had injected Novacaine into her thumb so at least I wasn't hurting her. In fact, she was very patient and calm, and never questioned my floundering but intense attempts. As a final resort I had to call the Old Man down. He looked at it briefly, then grabbed a pair of pliers and drove the hook deeper into her thumb and out the other side, snipped off the exposed barb and slipped the hook back out the original puncture site all in 30 seconds. The girl thanked me for taking the hook out. I felt ridiculous for getting the credit in spite of my incompetence!

We reminisced about our Newfoundland summer that was nearing an end. It wasn't the medical atmosphere that either one of us wanted in the future, but we felt fortunate to have experienced a type of medical practice that was rapidly fading from existence. Training at Strong Memorial or Mass General was all about medicine—on this tiny island it was all about the patient. The direct interaction between a doctor and his patient on this desolate island seemed so unique. I didn't have malpractice insurance when I walked into the house that night and injected morphine into the bloodstream of a dangerously ill old man. I didn't do much, but my actions could have been worse than nothing if I had killed him with too much morphine. Hell, he could have died on his own without my helping him, but I had very little to lose and the reward was more than tea and cod.

And we didn't have culture plates or a microbiology lab to determine specific antibiotics for specific organisms. I didn't draw daily blood for esoteric blood tests, and chest x-rays were reserved for definite indications rather than done routinely as part of a hospital admission work-up. Without sophisticated inhalation-therapy equipment, anti-static boots or special duty nurses, somehow the patients survived and I could see no significant disproportion in mortality rates between this Newfoundland outpost and the University hospital where I had trained for 3 years. Sure, a very small percentage of patients have special problems that benefit from the medical heroics possible only in well-endowed hospitals. Fortunately, medicine is advancing to the point where it can favorably treat this minority. But for the great majority of patients, good basic medical practice is sufficient. What is harmful is to be avoided, what is curative is to be initiated, and what is irrelevant or redundant is to be eliminated. Vital to implementing all three of these principles is the ability to observe.

Mike drove me back to the hospital because it was my day on call.

Sunday was unusually quiet so I would have time to make leisurely ward rounds and settle down to some good reading. The first bit of news I got was that the Mountie had been up and wanted me to call him as soon as possible. Oh, God—what have I done now? With a sense of sick resignation that rapidly removed my need for a donut and coffee I picked up the phone and called his headquarters. Much to my relief, the only thing wrong was Constable Scott's stomach. It seemed that he awakened with a severe headache and nausea and then vomited twice. His stomach continued to hurt so would I please come down to check on him? Well, Mike had the van but I wasn't about to wave that red flag in front of constable. So I asked him to pick me up as the van was "being used at the moment".

Meanwhile, I went to get my instruments and some pills that might be helpful. But the more I thought, the more coincidental the situation seemed. It was Sunday noon—did that have any bearing on Constable Scott's aching belly or was it purely coincidental that last night was Saturday night? It could be a flu-type illness causing gastroenteritis, but diarrhea is often present and there was no mention of that. So I threw in some Compazine and Maalox and walked down the road to meet my ride.

Constable Scott was having his problems. As I walked into his quarters, he was lying on one elbow staring at a basin he held in his hand. His face gave away the diagnosis at first glance—bloodshot eyes, coated tongue, hang dog expression. I asked him a few questions and examined his belly. A quick listen and a few pushes caused him to wretch, but nothing came up. He flopped back on his pillow in exhaustion. The diagnosis of a good stiff hangover was so obvious that it was embarrassing, and the Mountie suggested that it might have been some bad meat that he had eaten last night. I said no, I didn't think so, but that I had some pills to make him feel better. We all understood each other very well though nothing explicit was mentioned. The next day he brought up a medical form to be filled out. This was required for any treatment administered to a Mountie, and it had to be forwarded to the central office in Toronto. I got down to the key line where it asked for the diagnosis, hesitated for a moment to feel him squirm as he looked on and jotted down "mild gastroenteritis". He quietly thanked me for the pills that had made him feel so much better, shook my hand and left. Mike and I were golden.

That afternoon in clinic Al beckoned me to his office. He had the young woman with petit mal epilepsy with him for a follow-up visit. She was very attentive and seemed to be doing quite well on Tridione. I appreciated his gesture. Fortunately clinic was short that day, uncommon for a Monday. I had planned to check up on Mr. Jenkins, the 80 year-old man I had admitted for pulmonary edema, and then sack out for a while. Mike told me I had a letter in my box, so I stopped by on the way to the ward. It was from Kathleen and must have come by way of row boat judging from the date on the postmark. She lived on another island so that explained part of it. She told me she was feeling fine and had no more right mid-back pain. Then a lot of little news which included the fact that they did not have a teacher for the fall and it looked as if she would not be going to school that year. She finished the letter by inviting me to her home if I could ever come, saying that her father wanted to meet me. She signed it, "Your patient, Kathleen".

It was a nice letter. I folded it up and put it in my back pocket and lifted out my stethoscope as I walked to the ward. Mr. Jenkins' chest still had a few rales but clinically he was about 80% better. His chest x-ray had cleared considerably and the EKG showed the digitalis effect on the S-T segment. His only complaint was a slight pain in his right calf muscle. I couldn't see any swelling or redness and he was inconsistent in his response to my squeezing the calf. I elevated his legs on pillows as a precaution against stagnant blood clotting in his veins.

Mike had the duty that night so I turned in early. We had an agreement not to turn the light on when the other guy was sleeping so I got a little upset when he barged in and flipped it on.

"Hey, turn the damn light off, huh?"

"Dick, Jenkins died." He announced. "Don't know what it was. The nurse called me and he was dead."

I told Mike about Jenkins' problems with his right leg. It was possible that a blood clot had formed in his leg, dislodged, and then settled in a major lung artery—a fatal pulmonary embolus. He also could have had a heart attack but without an autopsy, I was only speculating. Autopsies were not done in Twillingate.

If it had been an embolus then I had underestimated the significance of his leg pain. I thought I had been sufficiently observant, but perhaps I hadn't been observant enough. I would never know.

CHAPTER TWENTY

THE ONE THAT GOT AWAY

"Turbulence is life force. It's opportunity."
William Ramsey Clark, U.S. Attorney General

"Whole Lotta Shakin' Goin' On",
Jerry Lee Lewis, 1957

An interesting phenomenon prevalent in the Newfoundland waters throughout the summer is a complex
predator-prey cycle. Early in June lobsters are usually
abundant, feeding among the protective shoals and fatten-
ing up for the mating season. Some seasons are a sparse
producer of this highly prized marine crustacean, though
the factors that affect year-to-year variations are not obvious.

In late June and early July the capelin swarm to the
shores to spawn. This is a vulnerable time for many
species, especially so for the capelin. Their process of
spawning is intense and attention getting, many of them so
fatigued by their efforts that they are easy prey for anything
from crabs to humans. This cornucopia greatly benefits
flounder, who hunt individually, and the huge schools of
cod. The cod, in turn, are an easy target for the jiggers and
nets, and provide the main product for the fishing indus-
try. Then in late August the big bluefin tuna move in,
feeding on the cod and smaller fish, often chasing them
deep into inland channels.

Newfoundland bluefin are abundant. People charter tuna boats for $80-$100 a day with the guarantee that they will at least see tuna if not hook one. One August, the St. John's radio boasted that the tuna seen that day were so plentiful you could walk across Bonavista Bay on the backs of the bluefins. Mike and I were invited to go tuna fishing on several occasions.

Our first excursion was on a 24 foot inboard craft and it was an all day affair. Paul, the skipper, was a self-made Newfie success story, a true Horatio Alger type. Raised on the island, he went to high school and then struck out on his own. He started a small shop with appliances, then added radios and built a second shop in Gander; then a third in St. Johns where he rapidly expanded to include color TV sets, stereo equipment and the like. He was a prodigious reader, and had a library that included books on lung physiology and tuberculosis, genetics, architecture, Chinese art, the French and Italian Renaissance, geology and oceanography. He was a big playmate to his two sons, and had a beautiful 3-level house. Practical and aggressive, he stood 6 foot 2 inches, weighed 250 pounds, and was always in motion, purposeful motion.

During winter he was a guide for hunting moose in his spare time and was always building something or working on a new project. Paul drove the only Cadillac I ever saw in Newfoundland, a gold 1964 El Dorado convertible. He was self-assured, outspoken and clever and got along well with everyone, especially Johnny Walker Red.

The dual inboard engines drove us at 20 knots directly out to sea for a mile, then up the coast. He was an old hand at this, but had never fished for tuna in waters this far north. He claimed that the vast majority of tuna caught in

Newfoundland were 500 pounds or more. The bigger tuna were more apt to swim near the surface for their food and could more successfully compete against the slower and smaller tuna. One tuna weighing about 1300 pounds had been caught commercially, but the record for a private catch was in the 900's. Anyone catching a tuna over 1000 pounds was made an honorary citizen of Newfoundland and got a prize of $1 a pound.

Finding bluefin tuna is keyed to their feeding habits. They swim in huge schools of 200 to 300 in search of food. Their small prey, unable to go deep, are forced to the surface. It is here that the massacre occurs and the surface boils with activity. Seagulls are always on hand as scavengers, sandwiching the smaller fish between them and the tuna. Green black water churns into a white, frothy display in an intense fight for survival. The patch of scarred ocean moves progressively and orderly across the surface as the huge lumbering tuna relentlessly keep pace with their frantic prey. Giant triangular fins smoothly slice the surface, undisturbed by the screams and dives of crazed gulls who greedily share in the feast. The gulls' flight pattern is the most sensitive indicator of any change in direction of the smaller fish. The gulls may suddenly veer off one way or the other, reflecting a new orientation of the prey in their desperate attempt to escape. Slowly this new orientation becomes evident in the water itself where the tuna drive off in fresh pursuit.

From a distance only the gulls could be seen, appearing as small white specks through binoculars. The engines responded, throwing us against the bulkhead as Paul applied full throttle. The specks grew larger until we saw their dives and heard their screams. The tuna were submerged but we paralleled the chase and could make out their huge blue black forms which slipped so effortlessly through the water and dove in slow motion style beneath our boat as we cut across the periphery of the school.

My heart pounded with focused intensity as I sat in the swivel chair eagerly anticipating what 500 pounds of force would feel like in my inexperienced hands. The chair was a unit composed of a wooden seat with two metal bars supporting a sturdy foot rest. The unit pivoted on a single supporting post so the seat could revolve 360 degrees. I sat with my feet on the cross bar, but otherwise was in no way attached to the seat or the boat. I wore a heavy harness with metal clips that fastened to the sides of the huge reel, and the thick rod rested in a hole in the seat between my legs. This arrangement provided a mechanical advantage where leverage spared the arms and utilized the legs. If I forced my legs out against the foot rest and simultaneously arched my back, the rod would be forced back with me because of the harness, as the drag on the tuna increased. Quickly releasing from this position resulted in a small amount of slack in the line, quickly taken up by reeling in. The legs and back thus take up all the strain, leaving the arms free for reeling slack line. The struggle often lasted two or more hours, and a man's arms could not hold up for that long.

I sat in the chair as Mike carefully inserted the huge steel hook into the bait's mouth and deftly drew the tip out through its belly. The hook was connected to twelve feet of steel wire leader, which in turn was fastened to twenty feet of doubled 130 pound test line, followed by 800 yards of 130 pound test line. The extra strength of the wire leader and doubled line prevented it from breaking when the tuna was in close and could exert more force.

We paralleled the direction of the tuna, slowly advancing to about 50 yards in front and to the side of them. I was unaware of the engines, the gas fumes, the sea spray, the screaming gulls. All I thought of was what the explosive pull would feel like and how I hoped I would respond. I paid out 70 yards of line and the skipper angled the boat diagonally across the incoming tuna. It was a strange sensation to see this mass of fin and fish coming toward us point blank. What would happen if I fell overboard? Reflexively, I drove my feet hard against the cross bar. The bait, ahead of the tuna, caused a small but visible mini wake. A bluefin broke suddenly and angled for it and we sped up to stimulate his chase. The tuna hit like hell. There was a brief but tremendous silent surge on the rod which drew on my tense arms and back, then the scream of the reel as the drag was overcome and the tuna dove for deep water. Reverberations of bluefins inadvertently striking the line could be felt as he dove between them, but the line held and the reel screamed its triumph.

The line assumed a deeper and deeper angle with the water as the tuna dove, but the reel's drag and the high pressure of deep water slowed his descent, though he remained at this depth for well over 30 minutes. I burned my fingers on the reel trying to readjust the drag and found it much more sensible to use a rag. Even more sensible would have been to have worn gloves. By increasing the drag, the tuna had to fight much harder in order to run, and I had to strain more to hold him. As the tension on the line reached dangerously high levels, I relaxed the drag to let him run a bit until he tired. Then I would increase the drag and reel in foot by foot. All this going on with the boat at 10 knots or so to keep pace with the tuna. As the gulls altered their course so we altered out course in relation to the tuna's direction, trying always to keep him directly astern.

My muscles burned continuously, with occasional interruptions of sharp brief stabs of pain, and I had to change position and slowly twist my back for some relief. Aware of the purpose of my discomfort, it felt good. I finally pulled him to the doubled line and made out a shiny, immense black form briefly before he spied the boat and ran again. I sensed he was tiring to the point where I could increase the drag and literally haul him through the water. He slowly lumbered to the surface and gently broke the water 100 yards away, and I knew he was mine.

Twenty-five minutes later I had reeled him into the double line again with the drag set very high. I was overanxious and under-experienced and had grossly underestimated his reserve. Suddenly, I felt a quick tremendous pull on the line which yanked me out of my chair and slammed me against the stern of the boat. For a brief instant I pictured myself, rod, reel and all, catapulting over the stern and being dragged into deep water. Before that flash of fear subsided, the line had snapped and I fell back onto the deck. The slack line whipped freely about in the wind and I felt intense defeat.

Everything had been so full and now was so empty.

Everything that had felt so good now hurt like hell.

The sweet, steady pull had been such a constant reminder of my victory; I had assumed it would last, but it hadn't, and its loss was now so final.

I felt idiotic, sprawled unceremoniously on the deck and unhooked myself from the harness. Everyone shared my disappointment. But now it was Mike's turn and there were still more tuna than we had a right to see. Mike had equal luck in getting a beautiful strike. Apparently learning from my over-zealous mistake, he used more patience in playing him. The fight lasted exactly two hours, and though I envied him sitting there, it was a more relaxing chance to observe the maneuvers and behavior of tuna. They go deep first and fight on and on until they tire. Then they surface but never leap or tail fin as do marlin. They have tremendous reserves of strength and the only way to succeed is to outlast them.

Mike outlasted his tuna and was reeling in double line with steel leader shining its way into the tuna's mouth. The skipper took a large gaff hook in his gloved hand and easily sunk it deep into the underbelly. He pulled up enough to lift the tuna's head out of the water and the fight was over. He was too large to haul aboard so the skipper passed a heavy line through his mouth and gills and we towed him home. Mike was the local hero, and the next day a crowd gathered for the weighing. A heavy rope was secured around the large, Y-shaped tail fin and the fish was slowly lifted up from the boat. The tip of the nose inched away from the deck as the crane assumed the entire weight of this creature. 607 pounds dry weight, plus 10% for water loss. Total—667 pounds. Since there was no market here for fresh tuna, Mike had it cut up into steaks and frozen. Each member of the hospital staff received a box of these steaks, and there was some for the constables and plenty more to go around.

I went after tuna twice more, both times getting a strike and both times losing it. The second time was a gray, drizzling day and we had to give up early. The drab, treeless coast was camouflaged by mist and rain as we headed back, our trip aggravated by swells of a quartering sea which monotonously rocked us between crest and trough. Once inside the protection of the outer harbor the water smoothed out, ruffled only by an occasional cats' paw, and figures began to emerge through the mist. By the time I could make out a dory, dozens of others came into sight, two men to a dory, each with a line in hand which they jerked up and down quickly. This was squid jigging time, and judging from the excitement and action, the waters were rich in this prized catch.

We dropped anchor to join in the haul. The skipper put on a foul weather suit while he assured me I would be all right in my dungarees and pullover college sweater, which fortunately was old and ready to go anyhow—though I had used it for everything from a sailing windbreaker to a ski jacket and guarded it like an old dog. He produced two 4-inch-long squid jigs which looked like the metal framework of an old umbrella. The central stem was bright red and the small, curved metal spines ended in a sharp tip without barbs. Red is the fighting color of squid as it is for other animals such as the robin, back fish and bull, and squid are compulsively, physiologically responsive to this stimulus. There is no choice in the matter, and a squid's extreme aggressiveness is an impressive phenomenon.

I suspended the jig from a line and gaped at its descent into the black water. At precisely 6 feet a circular surge of squid jetted to the jig, and my reactive surprise resulted in two squid. They easily slipped off the smooth spines onto the deck, and while captivated by their squirming efforts, I was jerked from concentration by a shock of stinging wet, foul tasting squid ink which at once filled my eyes and mouth. This squid juice helps the squid escape from a predator by propelling the squid away at a fast speed. More importantly, it leaves the predator in a literal black cloud of dust, rendering the squid invisible as he darts away from the danger zone.

Captain Paul had just introduced me to the art of "squid squirting" wherein one grabs the bloated squid and squeezes vigorously, resulting in a forceful blast of squid ink. The Captain gave me another shot of squid juice directly in my face, the black, viscous, gooey material clung to my eyebrows and dribbled down my cheeks, blurring my vision just long enough to allow him another opportunity to blast me again.

By the time I had cleared my eyes, spit in disgust and retaliated I was already behind 3 to 1. It was a non-stop battle lasting 30 minutes or more, and I ended up black and slimy as the deck. We slipped on squished squid, laughed at each others' antics and became adept at down the neck and up the nose shots. The amount of squid never dwindled—- we began to feel the cold and decided to head in. Just a couple of guys having fun!

CHAPTER TWENTY ONE

FAREWELL TO TWILLINGATE

*"A true friend is someone who thinks that
you are a good egg even though he knows
you are slightly cracked."*
Bernard Meltzer, radio host

"Days of Wine and Roses",
Henry Mancini, 1963

The night before I left Newfoundland, Mike and I threw a party for the entire hospital and a few scattered locals including the two dismounted Mounties. A lot of preparation had gone into this party, both in home grown decorations as well as procuring food. The nurses had done a great job in hanging streamers and fake flowers, and Mike's personal touch was a huge, multi-colored sign which read, "Dick is leaving. What better reason for a celebration!"

Our crowning glory—the food came from the sea. Grilled tuna steaks which tasted like the best swordfish I had ever had; contraband, out-of-season lobster which everyone enjoyed immensely; capelin, a bit dry and too salty but good with lots of beer; small snails that we had to pick out with safety pins and dip into spicy sauce; sautéed squid which was a bit rubbery but exotic; delicious flounder and not so delicious cod of which I had had my fill by now—all washed down with either beer or Newfie screech, another indiscreet transgression which the constables generously overlooked and even more generously helped themselves.

It really was a fantastic party though I'm afraid patient care suffered a bit that night. Mike had the duty and a man from the fishery came in with a badly cut hand. Mike stumbled down to the clinic while we continued to party. Ten minutes later he stumbled back reporting, "The damn thing didn't need any stitches. Anyway, I couldn't see to sew it up. Give me a beer."

Perhaps by University hospital standards, patient care in our hands suffered a bit all summer. We were lacking both knowledge and experience and did not have the benefits of academically rigorous, sophisticated medicine. But I think for that very reason, because we were made very aware of our relative inadequacies, we were stimulated to challenge our methods and decisions to a greater degree. We asked each other questions, ran to our books constantly, squeezed the meager lab facilities to the limit, and learned to take x-rays when the tech was on holiday.

It was this direct involvement that was so satisfying. A man came into the clinic with an injured arm. I examined him, took an x-ray, developed and read the x-ray, diagnosed a fracture and applied a cast. In a University hospital this one case would involve six people—the desk secretary, liaison nurse, surgical intern, x-ray tech, radiologist and the orthopedic surgeon to apply the cast.

It was great to assume total responsibility and not have to garner fragments of information or help from six different sources. This was the best part of the summer's experience—to be in a position to assume responsibility, to make independent decisions, to sweat out potential complications of my method of treatment, to criticize and scrutinize why I was surprised when things went right, and why I wasn't when things went wrong. I had done my first tonsillectomy and hernia, sutured a severed tendon in less than orthodox fashion but with satisfactory results in terms of healing and function; made a diagnostic coup with the infant who had pyloric stenosis and been asked to read an EKG, which at my level of training would have been absurd in an academic environment, and yet, at this small hospital, perhaps was not so absurd.

Twillingate forced on me demands of a different type from those of med school, a direct physical immersion into medicine, doing more than I deserved or had the ability to do. And now I was headed back into a compulsive, highly academic program where, because of the rightful emphasis on the highest degree of knowledge, fragmentation, specialization, and esoteric tests and examinations were the rule—a sharp contrast with the encompassing responsibility of that summer.

I thought about these things many times while walking the hospital corridors and ordering these very esoteric tests. Twillingate had given me a tangible basis on which to challenge rather than accept, and by comparison to realize the significance of appropriate medical care in radically different settings. One has to be appropriate, and I sobered to this realization during the years to come, but I tried to keep with me the ingenuity and resourcefulness behind treating that old Newfie with belts and pillows.

When I said goodbye to the Old Man, I found him between cases, sitting as usual in green scrubs, gown and gloves, mask hanging down and curling a deep inhale of pipe smoke from his mouth. He pre-empted me as soon as I opened my mouth to speak. "Richard, you have a lot of potential. Once you overcome being tentative, you will hit your stride. Have confidence in your abilities".

I had a parting comment all prepared in my mind but he put down his pipe, turned and walked back into the OR. I shot out, "Thank you, sir," but I'm not even sure he heard it.

Al drove me to the Gander airport. We bumped across the gap onto the ferry in his VW for the last time. I stood next to the car, leaning over the ferry railing, feeling the engine vibrations under my feet and watching the wake curl away from the ferry as Twillingate grew smaller in the distance. This had been an experience I knew I would never be able to duplicate. The rest of the drive was pretty much in silence. We arrived at the airport and we shook hands goodbye. Al looked sad. Nothing said, just sad. My plane lifted off and it was goodbye to Newfoundland.

A change of planes in Boston, and a few hours later I stepped off the plane and searched the people at the gate for the sight of my family. Lynn was jumping up and down waving at me; Carol smiled at me. Lynn ran and leaped into my arms. We hugged for a solid minute.

It was good to be home.

SECTION THREE:

FINISH LINE

CHAPTER TWENTY TWO

"FYBIGMI"

"No one can cheat you out of ultimate
success but yourself"
Ralph Waldo Emerson, American essayist

"Oh, How Happy!"
Shades of Blue (1966)

As an extern (fourth year medical student), I had the privilege of going down to the emergency room to screen patients for surgical evaluation. ER's are the same everywhere: patients in pain, anxious relatives, sometimes a policeman or a first responder, but in a teaching hospital, the young person in the green scrubs may or may not be a "real" doctor yet.

The ER at first appears chaotic: secretaries, doctors, and nurses all talking at once, either on the phone or to each other; papers everywhere, x-rays in clumps on the viewing box, EMT's, police and fireman in the hallway or stuffing down some leftover chocolate cake or stale pizza with jet black coffee from the nurse's station while the OR staff loaded and wheeled an emergent patient to the OR on a gurney. But bees in a hive seem chaotic too, yet every individual has a focused and distinct job to do. The kinetic motion and noise are simply accepted background against which labs are reviewed, patients seen, tests ordered and decisions made.

The structure of the ER looks something like this:

Triage the patient according to the nature of the presentation, i.e. routine, semi-emergent, or emergent. If emergent, then stabilize (IV fluids, plasma, blood, oxygen), diagnose (lab, EKG, radiographic studies, ultrasound), and treat. If non-emergent, diagnose and treat under less stressed conditions. Once the diagnosis is made, the appropriate specialist is summoned, i.e. pediatrician, internal med, cardiology, orthopedic, neurologist, urologist, surgeon, etc. Treatment will be either non-surgical (medications, fluid replacement, observation, etc.) or surgical—if surgical, it will be either immediate, delayed until another more urgent case is completed or scheduled for the next day.

Another category could be classified as malingerers. These are the patients who clog the system and gravitate to the ER out of convenience, demand for drugs ("Doctor, I'm hurting. Give me morphine". These patients always ask for their "drug d'jour" by name). Other patients are motivated by boredom, or hunger. Tragically, there is the disoriented "Gomer" who gets discarded by the frustrated family in the ER parking lot and wanders into the ER on his own.

A middle-aged, overweight woman, with stringy dirty blonde hair, lay prone on the gurney. The top of her faded blue floral print house dress looked chronically lived in. I glanced at her shoes on the floor. Scuffed flats with run down heels and stretched out sides could have been black fake leather when new. Like the stern, pitchfork grasping stoic Mid-West couple depicted in Grant Woods' painting "American Gothic", her husband stood next to her in deafening silence. His watery pale blue eyes stared straight ahead. Neither spoke. The husband nodded at me as I approached his wife. I introduced myself.

"Mr. Grimes, I'm Dr. German, the extern on call for the emergency room. How can I help you?"

Without addressing me by name, and avoiding eye contact, this tall, gangly somewhat disheveled and extremely taciturn man replied, "It's my wife. She has something wrong up here," as he pressed his right hand against his chest.

I smelled the pungent odor of rotting flesh permeating the bed sheets. Trying not to react to the smell, I pulled the sheets back to reveal a fungating, necrotic right breast stuck to her house dress. A circle of moisture stained the dress over the right breast. When I opened her dress, I saw that the entire breast had become distorted and blackened from the malignant tumor that had started as a small pea-sized growth deep within her breast. As the tumor progressively grew through multiple mitotic divisions, it distorted the architecture of the breast. The cancer had penetrated the nipple and skin, both of which became indistinguishable in a mass of green-black necrotic, friable tissue that disintegrated under mild palpation. The breast, or what remained of it, was totally insensitive, and the woman felt no pain as I gently dislodged fragmented and bleeding chunks of tumor to send to pathology for definitive diagnosis.

As I proceeded, the woman glanced at her husband. Either he wasn't aware of her apparent need for reassurance, or he was aware and did not care, because he did not reciprocate. After every unanswered request for comfort, the woman's small hazel eyes watered a little more. Her husband continued to stare across her body at a point in space beyond the gurney.

"Mrs. Grimes? How long have you been aware of this condition?" I asked my patient.

When she didn't answer, I looked at her and saw her staring at her husband as if expecting him to supply the information.

"Arthur?" Apparently this stoic woman was totally subordinate to her dour husband. "Please..."

"She stank for some time," he said before clearing his throat. "Can't do nothing no more."

It became obvious she had no say in her own health status. Apparently, he sought medical attention for his wife because of the intolerable odor of her disease process, her reduced capacity to perform household duties, and the subsequent increased demands on his time.

Unbelievably, the work-up showed no metastatic involvement of her lungs, bones or liver, so we prepared her for surgery the next day. She was scheduled for a radical mastectomy to include removal of the entire breast, both chest wall muscles (pectoralis major and minor) and complete axillary lymph node dissection.

Since I had done the intake, I was assigned as first assistant for her surgery. Her dirty blond hair beneath a transparent gauze shower cap, her right arm extended on an arm board, she was positioned on the OR table. An IV and blood pressure cuff were on her left arm and the patient was anesthetized and intubated. The nurse prepped the operative site—the entire right breast and chest wall, axilla and upper arm down to the elbow. It was strange to see the white soapy prep flushing over the tumor which then reappeared in its black, necrosing and bleeding form as the soap trickled between the crevices and dribbled off on to the sterile towels, like a foamy wave crashing over a chunk of conglomerate rock.

The surgeon applied the drapes so only the breast, axilla and upper arm were visible. He took a felt marking pen and traced out a large tear drop-shaped incision, the point starting high in the axilla, going widely around the entire breast on both sides and forming the bottom of the tear drop near the lower part of the sternum. The breast was covered with a sticky transparent Saran Wrap-type covering (steri-drape) to preserve tumor integrity and to avoid troublesome bloody fragments from being dislodged during the procedure.

"Knife, please..."

He took the knife from the scrub nurse and made a clean, sharp perpendicular incision through the skin starting at the sternum and following the black felt pen tracing. First he cut the lower (inferior) incision down through the dermis and subcutaneous tissue, then tapering through the deep tissue to insure removal of all breast tissue down to the rib cage. As first assistant, I retracted the skin margins and helped control bleeding. All necrotic and malignant tissue stayed well within the confines of the steri-drape and never came in contact with the surgeon's gloves. The principle is to remove all remaining normal breast tissue peripheral to the malignancy without contacting the malignancy itself. The deeper we cut the more vigorous the bleeding which was controlled by a combination of cautery, clamping and free hand 2-0 silk ties or 2-0 silk suture ligatures, all cut just above the knot (in order to minimize the volume of foreign material left in the surgical site).

The surgeon pinched off the bleeding vessel with the curved tip of the four-inch long Kelly clamp. The assistant is handed a fourteen-inch long black silk "free tie" (no needle attached) by the scrub nurse. She uses both hands, one on either end of the free tie and forcefully lifts it up to meet the outstretched hand (palm down) of the assistant. This is to insure that the assistant knows he has been handed a tie since his attention may well be, and often is, directed not at the nurse, but to the surgical field so as not to avert his eyes. His hand goes to the nurse for the tie, his eyes remain in the field for concentration and speed. He then passes the silk tie around the tip of the clamp being held by the surgeon, and places a single throw (half of the knot). The surgeon removes the clamp so the first throw can be further tightened around the tissue. The second throw is then placed, again by the assistant, insuring it is a perfect square knot that will not loosen. Finally, a third throw is placed, square to the previously placed knot and the suture cut just above the knot at a 45 degree angle to avoid cutting through the knot itself. When that happens, and it does, the tie unravels, bleeding resumes and the surgeon gives the "evil eye" to the assistant who incorrectly cut the suture. You are allowed one "evil eye" per case— end of story.

Once the inferior flap had been developed, the surgeon cut along the superior margin until we curved our way up to the tip of the tear drop in the axilla and met the rising margin from the previously dissected inferior flap. At this point we reflected (pulled upwards) most of the breast, but the deep central portion of the tumor had drilled its way into the underlying pectoralis major muscle. That was the next to go, and we progressively dissected the entire muscle away from the chest wall and rib cage attachments with the carefully applied cautery. The cautery, meant to coagulate the smaller veins and arteries, would occasionally sever larger diameter vessels which had sufficient pressure to shoot up a spray of blood onto our surgical face masks before we could clamp and tie them off.

A few sprinkles of blood splattered the surgeon's glasses and the float nurse quickly wiped them clean before driblets of blood, now contaminated by a non-sterile object (surgeon's glasses), could fall back down onto the sterile surgical field.*

The entire breast/tumor, pectoralis major and minor muscles were now reflected en mass up to the axilla, revealing a bare chest wall of only ribs and intercostal muscles. As the surgeon progressively divided the large pectoralis muscle groups from their attachment to the chest wall, I

---

* As an interesting side note, on rare occasion a devious fly will find its circuitous way from the outside world all the way down the hospital corridor into the operating room and torture the surgeon's attention. The protocol is as follows – all lights in the operating room are turned off (meanwhile the patient is fast asleep and the surgeon's hands are motionless in the surgical field. The only sounds are the sighs of the respirator rhythmically pumping anesthetic gas into the patient and the damn fly buzzing around); the scrub room door adjacent to the operating room is opened and the fly is attracted to the light wherein he is summarily executed. If by chance, and it has happened, the fly lands onto the operative field, attracted by the open wound and blood, the area must be re-prepped and draped immediately. If he lands on the sterile-instrument Mayo stand, all instruments must be replaced. From the surgeon's point of view, it is a colossal and frustrating waste of time, let alone a nasty potential for infection. Can you imagine the surgeon having to explain to the patient, "Mrs. Jones, I'm sorry for your wound infection but a fly landed on your open breast in the middle of the operation!" Most operations have their own moments of excitement—it is the responsibility of a competent surgeon to minimize and control those moments. Just like a pilot, a surgeon wants a boring, routine, straightforward operation with no surprises or heart pounding events.

clamped the supporting vessels and small nerves and then divided then with a momentary and final neurologic twitch in the muscle being removed.

Dissection of the many lymph nodes from the axilla, 15 to 20 of them, was the last and most dangerous part of the procedure. They might contain possible micro-metastases from the parent breast tumor, all lying close to the axillary vein and artery, and nestled dangerously close to the profound complex of nerves called the brachial plexus (providing motor power and sensation to the entire upper extremity). Injure or sever any of those structures and the surgeon has a monumental and sometimes irreversible problem on his hands, not to mention the patient who may end up with a partially paralyzed arm. This is what the surgeon is trained for: to completely remove and dissect out all the lymph nodes in an uneventful manner.

The surgeon started this final stage of lymph node dissection in the usual manner, by first identifying the big, blue axillary vein where it leaves the upper arm and enters the axilla laterally. Dissection then progressed in a lateral to medial direction along the border of the vein, teasing the lymph nodes away from the vessels and brachial plexus. My job was to isolate the tiny supporting veins, doubly clip them with small 2 to 4 mm stainless steel hemoclips, and divide without tearing the delicate axillary vein or molesting the unforgiving bifurcating nerve bundle of the brachial plexus. High up in the axilla, and running down the lateral chest wall over the ribs was the subtle but discrete long thoracic nerve. To confirm its identity, the surgeon gently pinched the nerve with long forceps. We watched her shoulder jump vigorously. The nerve enervates the muscles supporting the scapula and inadvertent division (an unforgivable technical error) of the nerve results in corresponding muscle paralysis and a permanent condition known as winged scapula. The scapula, or shoulder blade, would flop helplessly away from the upper back and look like a permanent wing—an atrocious and cosmetically disastrous result.

The surgeon completed the dissection without incident (no complication) and inserted two large polyethylene tubes 4mm in diameter against the rib cage and under the skin to drain serum and blood from deep in the wound. The dense dermis was brought together with multiple interrupted sutures, and the skin finally closed with stainless steel staples.

Skin to skin (incision to closure)—2 hours 18 minutes.

Case over.

The patient did well post-op, recovered and went home. I felt so badly for her. She seemed so emotionally beaten down and hardly spoke during her hospitalization, even for pain meds. Her husband came in once, to pick her up. I never saw her again, not even in the post-op outpatient clinic. I suspect she was back to cooking and making the bed so as not to inconvenience her husband.

And the rest of the story....

Fourth year med school flew by. There was no question in my mind that I wanted to become a surgeon and all my efforts focused on this goal. The other required disciplines (e.g., pediatrics, internal medicine) were behind me and I could concentrate on the intensity of the OR. I could finally see the light at the end of the tunnel.

Each med student lists his choice of internship on a computerized form as does each hospital its choice of students, and by a matching process, internships are assigned. Students make their choice based on geographic and academic preference. The hospitals base their choice purely on the academic standing of the student and recommendations given by their professors.

On a single magic day in mid-March, every med student in the country receives notification of where he will spend the next year (or more) of his life. The word goes out at mail time and every fourth year student makes tracks like tracer bullets to the mailroom—a casual observer or disliked professor is at risk of being trampled at this moment. This should be Webster's definition of focused energy.

For most there is elation and relief; for some, temporary disappointment.

Regardless, that evening the students will celebrate their accomplishments with a raucous rehearsed spoof in the same auditorium where we spent half our lives taking notes and exams. The professors were all there to take their lumps and we held very little back. This was known as "FYBIGMI Day", or "F—You, Buddy, I Got My Internship", the basic message to our superiors being "stop shitting on me and ordering me around, since I'll be out of here in three months."

Keep in mind the pecking order: third year med student—brain dead, pupils dilated; fourth year med student—some brainwave pattern developing, pupils responsive to light; intern—partially functioning, dangerous and capable of injuring patients; resident—uses scalpel to cut your balls off; chief resident—God.

The interaction between scalpel wielding resident and the student with partial brain activity is often demeaning and tiresome. So when the order comes down to repeat the rectal exam on a 90 year-old with chronic diarrhea, the proper response at this point is "FYBIGMI". Unless, of course, "God" asks you to do it.

The last internal med rotation was bittersweet. Bitter since this was my final exposure to intensive and sophisticated discussions of esoteric disease processes as presented by the internal med house staff, and critiqued by the brilliant Chief of Internal Medicine, Dr. Cassidy. In his mid-50's, tall and thin, graying hair, a perfectly trimmed moustache, his attire reflected his commitment to his calling. Brooks Brothers custom tailored pin striped suit, bright white perfectly pressed shirt, with a regimental tie set the stage for his penetrating intellect. When he spoke, we listened. With the precision of an incision, Dr. Cassidy's every word counted. Intuitive, informative, and important his presentations were recorded in our notebooks. Our notebooks became a convenient source of knowledge to be regurgitated at the appropriate time in the future. I knew I'd miss the intellectual stimulation unique to his service.

The sweet part? Surgery—the discipline of my dreams—was straight ahead in my future.

However, I had the month of May on Dr. Cassidy's service to wrap up my fourth year of medical school prior to my graduation at the end of the month. The senior resident, junior resident, intern and I made rounds on Dr. Cassidy's patients every day, as well as other unassigned patients who had been admitted through the ER. Occasionally Dr. Cassidy would lead us on rounds, often yielding lengthy discussions at the patient's bedside. If the subject was "touchy", i.e., cancer, terminal illness, bad prognosis, we held our discussions in the hallway out of the patient's earshot. Some things need not be discussed by a bunch of sober faces in starched white lab coats within hearing distance of the object of the discussion.

One day we were rounding on a diabetic patient who had been stabilized on insulin and was ready, in our opinion, for discharge. The senior resident directed the intern to write the order for discharge in the chart, and provide prescriptions for use at home, with an appointment for follow-up in the diabetic clinic. For every patient we saw, prior to hearing the disposition from above, I came up with my own conclusion as to further treatment. Discharging this diabetic patient seemed appropriate, and in my naïve thinking, I felt Dr. Cassidy would rubber stamp our discharge order.

Au contraire. Late that afternoon, I heard my name over the intercom to convene in Dr. Cassidy's office, "STAT". Meeting in his outer office, the four of us glanced at each other, adjusted out ties, hitched up our pants, and rubbed the dust off of our shoes on the backs of the opposite legs before filing through the door to his office...that he held open. Not a good sign.

He quietly closed the door behind us. Without a word of greeting, he walked to his desk. Instead of sitting in his leather chair, he deliberately moved a stack of manila folders to the side. Without looking up, he placed his knuckles on the blotter in front of him as he leaned over his desk. Scanning the four of us with intelligent green eyes, like a cat selecting which catnip mouse to pounce on, Dr. Cassidy waited ten to fifteen seconds before clearing his throat to ensure he had our focused attention on what he was about to say.

"The patient, this patient is my patient." He stood up as if his spine had solidified in cement. Another scan of the assembled "doctors", another throat clearing, and another extended pause.

I didn't know about the rest of them, but I felt my knees weaken just a little. I didn't dare look at the "senior" doctors on either side of me. It was enough, for this time, that I was the junior man on this particular totem pole.

"My patient." His voice softened, which had the intended effect of his students leaning forward in anticipation. "My patient."

Another scan of his students, and this time I could sense the "flop sweat" beading beneath the armpits of my associates.

"Do NOT discharge one of my patients without my knowledge or permission." Another scan, and by this time we were all examining the toes of our loafers. "Ever."

We risked looking up.

"He has insulin dependent diabetes," Dr. Cassidy continued, "He is not ready for discharge until I say he is ready for discharge."

I heard shuffling.

"Do I make myself clear?"

No response.

I thought I heard someone's stomach growl.

Maybe it was mine.

"You do understand that," Another pause. "Doctors?" He pronounced that word as if it were in quotes.

"Yes, sir." We mumbled, before filing out of his office.

Three days passed before I had the guts to ask the junior resident what had happened.

"It's economics, Rich." He said, pushing his Buddy Holly glasses up on his nose with the end of his ball point pen. "All economics".

"What about the patient's diabetes?" I asked.

"Don't be naïve. All of the attending physicians get paid a base salary. And they match their salary in private patient billing." He said with a tolerant sigh. "It doesn't matter what department they're in—surgery, ortho, OB-GYN, pediatrics, psychiatry, even radiology. It's the administration's way of rewarding them without having to up their salaries. So patient billing pays half of their income, the hospital the other half. Obviously, the attending surgeons get paid a lot quicker."

"So by keeping the patient in the hospital a day or two longer, Dr. Cassidy assures himself an income?"

"Bingo."

"Uh, huh." I grunted, not really knowing how to react to this information. Idealistic as are most med students, I couldn't quite justify extending patient care unnecessarily to "pad the bill". It occurred to me that I had a lot to learn in order to become a professional. Perhaps that's why doctors are known to be lousy businesspersons, and worse pilots. The practical applications of being a professional often escape us when we are pursuing our dream.

"Rich, it's all legal, well recognized and done everywhere. It increases the bill so that they get part of that money." He coughed. "Some of the attendings are more uptight than others when it comes to this issue."

"Oh," I said, trying to absorb...ok, justify the economics of my profession.

"Hey, no sweat for you——surgeons don't worry, because the operations cost enough to match their salary. Get with the program."

Years later (20 years or so) this was called "over-utilization" and the insurance companies rebelled. The higher the bill, the more money the insurance company paid out, and the less profit. So they raised their insurance premiums.   Then the patients, or their employers, squawked. Finally, the insurance company found the path of least resistance. They decreased the reimbursement to the doctors who took it on the chin and to the hospitals that resisted taking it on the chin. The hospitals, as much as they needed doctors, forced better and more appropriate utilization from its physicians. Taken to the extreme, insurance companies now pay a fixed amount of money for a particular hospital/physician service or operation. Thus it is in the physician's and hospital's best interest to discharge the patient at the earliest possible time—less is more.

But I trained during the glory (i.e. irresponsible) days, when more was more. No one had the foresight to predict the wages of our over-billing sins, to see the burden it placed on our health care system, to anticipate and alter the end of the gravy train. And these myopic individuals were the pillars of our medical and surgical programs, supposedly the smartest and best, and the crème de la crème. It took a tighter and tighter squeeze to initiate change, by which time economics imposed a radically new system on those brilliant but greedy physicians who lost the power to captain their own ship.

Suddenly, on a warm June day we wore the dark green sash signifying the discipline of medicine over our black gowns. Our names were called. We marched to the podium for the handshake and diploma. It took a few seconds, but represented a sobering commitment of time and energy for Lynn, Carol, me and our parents whose support contributed to the accomplishment.

My parents drove up from Connecticut with Oma, my dear Dutch grandmother. I think my Dutch determination came from Oma who held my hand as we walked across campus. She told me how proud she was.

Finally, I was gainfully employed! No more trash collecting, snack bar sales, house painting, morgue watch, or blood selling...real money for a real job...or so I thought.

I had matched to the surgical program at the University of Rochester.

Graduating from college had been rather anti-climatic, sort of "another day in the life". At that time I was married, had a 9 month-old daughter and faced ten more years of education and training—four years med school, one year internship and 5 years residency. Graduating from medical school had its own rewards: —at least I was an M.D. with the prospect of a paycheck. I sold my monocular microscope to a nursing home for $50—exactly what I had paid four years earlier. I gave up my part-time job as a trash collector and we moved into nicer digs at the University complex next to the hospital.

During my internship, walking home through 200 yards of deep snow during the upcoming five-month winter beat not getting home at all. Rochester had two seasons—winter and July. After four years it had grown monotonous and depressing.

CHAPTER TWENTY THREE

STAN THE MAN"

*"No plan has ever survived contact
with the enemy."*
General Napoleon Bonaparte

"You're the Devil in Disguise",
Elvis Presley, 1963

July 1, 1967—my first day as a paid physician, our first day as professionals, even though we were paid like indentured servants.

For my father who had circled that date in red on his calendar, July 1st, meant freedom from tuition payments. Thanks, Dad! Now, I was actually earning the princely sum of $300 per month and considering the hours, a parking meter would have been more profitable employment. Internship left no time or energy for moonlighting, and Carol and I faced a reduction in income from my extra work during med school. No time for the dog lab, garbage collecting, or selling my blood to the Red Cross for $25 a pint. Throughout med school, anemia was a constant concern. So when my blood count indicated approaching anemia, I picked up a little extra by working in the hospital morgue.

Knowing we were losing a percentage of our income was challenging, but without complaint Carol stepped up and continued as the real bread winner. We were working toward our future, and every time we looked at Lynn, we realized the importance of our efforts.

July 1st, 1967.
The time came for us to meet "God" face to face.
The first day of internship.
Ten of us, all men, all surgical interns, meeting for the first time, sat in the small conference room.

Then He walked in—the Chief Resident wearing scrubs and an attitude. He was about 5 feet 11 inches, slightly pudgy, balding yet handsome, with a 5 o'clock shadow at 8 a.m.

He spoke. "Welcome, gentlemen. I am Dr. Stan Moser, Chief Resident for the Surgical Service. A few rules: first, I don't want you spend time flipping through the hospital directory looking up numbers—memorize them; second, don't use the elevator (9 story medical center), use the stairs—it's quicker. If the elevator stops at every floor while your patient is arresting, the patient dies and you get replaced; third, eating and sleeping are luxuries—choose them carefully; fourth, when I need you, I need you; fifth, rounds start at 5:30 a.m. whether or not you are up all night in surgery. And when you assist me in surgery I expect silence and good retraction. That's it. Your supervising residents are ready to go over your patient assignments and responsibilities." With that he left and thereafter became known as "Malignant Stan".

I met my supervising resident, a euphemism for someone who had been as clueless as I had been twelve months before, yet somehow had survived, his ego very much intact. Shorter, plump, and infinitely superior to me, my resident was responsible for orienting the incoming surgical intern for his service. That would be me. He reminded me that I was only partially functioning, dangerous and capable of injuring patients.

Rounds done, he looked at me with a sober intensity and said, "I wouldn't be in your shoes for one million dollars." At that moment, he was paged overhead by the hospital operator. He picked up the wall phone.

"Yeah, what?" After a few seconds he continued. "Listen, just because it's July 1st and I'm now a first year resident doesn't mean life has changed much. I'll be home when I can". Even talking to his main support system, his own wife, I could tell what a toll the year had taken on their relationship.

Welcome to internship.

Our work schedule was 36 hours on, 12 hours off, which amounted to a 110 hour work week. At 68 cents an hour, the joke around the hospital: If you need more help, don't hire a nurse, hire an intern—he's cheaper.

A financially well off fellow intern was so insulted by the pay that he put his checks in a drawer to "screw up their accounting". In June when he left for another residency, he cashed all twelve checks. There are several types of internships: internal medicine, surgical, mixed med-surgical, pediatric, etc.

Thanks to my experience in Newfoundland, I knew with certainty that surgery was my specialty so I chose a straight surgical program. The interns rotated to a different surgical discipline every month—cardiovascular, plastic, general, urologic, ENT (ear, nose and throat), orthopedic, neurosurgery, thoracic, etc. The rotating interns had full exposure to all of the surgical disciplines in preparation for choosing their future specialty.

Cardiovascular and plastic gave me a tingle, general and neurosurgery definitely interested me, and the rest was a bore, especially ENT. My future would not be spent looking in ears, noses or throats.

Ironically, our ENT professor had a deformed nasal bridge that he had never corrected. One day during clinic, he demonstrated how to perform a minor nasal procedure under local anesthesia. He took two 8-inch long cotton tipped wires, dipped them into a tall jar of green liquid sitting on the shelf among tongue blades and cotton swabs. He then gently placed the two wires into the patient's nasal passage, cotton tip first, with no discomfort to the patient.

We left the room while the anesthetic took effect and discussed the planned procedure. When we returned a few moments later, the professor removed the wires and the patient had no nasal sensation.

What was that magic green solution?

Cocaine—pure, liquid cocaine, about 60 cc's worth sitting right up there on the shelf! We thought nothing of it at the time, but fast forward 20 years and that bottle would have disappeared faster than a jar of candy at a children's Christmas party.

Time spent in each surgical discipline was divided into making daily rounds on patients, spending time in the OR usually as second assistant, seeing new and post-op patients in the clinic, and doing "scut work" on the hospital floors (history and physical exams, drawing blood, checking on lab and x-rays, and writing pre-op orders.

Trial by Fire...

The Red Service (Cardiovascular) was brutal—up at 5 a.m. every day, rounding on all patients, scrubbing in for hours at a time, running down to see clinic patients, running back to the OR, performing late night exams, eating if possible and slipping into the ICU to catch a few hours of sleep on the cot if lucky enough to have a few hours between other responsibilities.

Plastic surgical rotation was the easiest. Almost all cases were elective and uncomplicated; low pressure rounds in the afternoon, clinic to follow, leisurely conference with the Junior and Senior Residents and home by 7 p.m.!

Thank God, my Red Service was the first (the month of July) on my schedule. From that point on it was easy riding by comparison—if working 110 to 120 hours a week can be easy!

What made things difficult was not the long working hours, but the pervasive back-East, uptight, rigid, Marine-like atmosphere, like a hydraulic press squeezing down on each level of house staff, from intern all the way up to Chief Resident. Aggravated by the "pyramid program", starting with twelve interns and ending up with only two Chief Residents, this pitted each level of resident against each other in pursuit of the Senior and Chief positions. Those residents who were not chosen for the next higher level were farmed out to other less competitive residency programs.

The Red Service required the interns to be indwelling, somewhat like a Foley catheter. Aptly named, the Red Service dealt in blood, blood and more blood, involving three disciplines:

1. <u>cardiac surgery</u> meant valve replacement and early coronary by-pass procedures. Both demanded going on pump, and new prosthetic valves and techniques were rapidly being developed;

2. <u>thoracic surgery</u> concentrated on the lungs, mainly trauma and tumors. The chest was a fun place to be—the anatomy was right in front of you, not hidden by bowel or liver; the surgery was clean, no bacteria or bowel contents inadvertently spilling into the wound; and the post-op infection rate was low—no wonder thoracic surgeons boast of their specialty "a day in the chest is like a year in the belly" (translation: the gratification of being a chest surgeon far, far exceeds that of being a general surgeon, at least in the eyes of a chest surgeon);

3. <u>vascular surgery</u> concentrated on the great vessels (aortic aneurysms), carotid arteries in the neck (blockage by arteriosclerotic plaque putting patients at risk of stroke) and femoral vessels (when blockage by plaque puts a patient's lower extremities at risk). Many vascular surgical procedures involved by-pass grafting. The graft material at that time was PTFE or polytetrafluoroethylene, a marvelous invention by Wilbert Gore. This material, better known as Gore-Tex, has had wide-spread applications, both inside as well as outside the human body. Mr. Gore hit a home run and his graft material has been used by surgeons the world over. And when the same surgeons go backpacking they wear waterproof Gore-Tex clothing and sleep in Gore-Tex tents.

There was only one surgical intern at a time on the Red Service. My duties were: take the history and perform the physicals on all new patients—everything was handwritten; write all pre-operative orders; confirm that lab and x-ray results were in the patient's chart; scrub in on cases assigned to me; have rounds on all patients done by 7:30 a.m. (which meant starting rounds by 5:00 a.m.); be available for emergency Red Service surgery anytime day or night; eat if necessary and sleep if possible. That meant curling up on a cot hidden behind a screen in the ICU, listening to the beeps of the EKG monitor while trying to fall asleep. If a patient suddenly arrested, I was 15 blurry seconds away from pounding on his chest and giving CPR.

Stamina required or do not apply.

The utter sense of physical exhaustion was overwhelming. Sleep deprivation mixed with psychological pressures to perform at peak levels can be a very debilitating stew, rattling the brain, sapping endurance and forcing the individual to seek sanctuary in self-preservation called sleep—sleep of variable duration, from minutes to several hours, but never, never enough to quench one's thirst.

I laid there on my uncomfortable, canvas cot, partially hidden by a flimsy, 5 foot tall metal framed curtain, impervious to the din of background ICU noise or the predictable glances of late shift nurses. I had an anemic hospital pillow and covered myself with a cheap, white multi-fenestrated OR blanket. The cot was so low that my hand rested on the floor, which surprisingly, was of comfort to me due to the vibrations of machines and personnel which transmitted the buzz of activity up my arm while I momentarily cheated the work load and rested supine.

The overhead fluorescent lights, scurry of feet, and rhythmic sighs of the respirators proved no competition for my fatigue. Not even the psychological bed of nails I was experiencing seemed to matter. My body was yielding inexorably to the enzymatic and physiologic drain on my conscious state. "I'm free at last, at least for the moment" and I rapidly feel into a deep sleep.

"Dr. German, Dr. German, Code Red in Bed 4"! The ICU nurse was bent over me, jiggling my shoulder vigorously. Adrenaline spurted out of my adrenal glands and into my bloodstream, fusing my heart and brain into instant response. I jerked out of my cot, ran to Bed 4, looked at the flat-line EKG monitor, and started CPR by placing the heel of my right hand over the back of my left hand and driving the sternum downward at one second intervals. This compressed the left ventricle into releasing its load of blood out into the aorta, up the carotid arteries and into the brain, a sensitive organ that abhors oxygen deprivation.

The clanging of a metal bedpan inadvertently kicked by a nurse against the IV pole was testimony to the chaos around me. All faded as just so much background noise. I was the boss—the doctor in charge, the pilot in control.

"1 amp of epi IV stat; power up the defibrillator; calcium, sodium bicarbonate now! Feel for a femoral pulse! Talk to me"! I was barking out orders like a Marine drill sergeant, but all to no avail. The patient remained flatlined with a rare erratic ventricular response—no V-tach (ventricular tachychardia) or V-fib (ventricular fibrillation) to cardiovert with the defibrillator. I remembered the words of my Chief: "If you apply cardioversion (electro shock) to a person with non-V-tach, V-fib erratic rhythm, you will cardiovert from an erratic rhythm to death."

Fifteen minutes of desperate CPR, continued flatline EKG and unresponsive dilated pupils, I pronounced the patient.

"CPR terminated, patient pronounced dead at 3:22 a.m. on this date, July 17, 1967. Notify the family."

I made a note in the chart to memorialize the events, wrote down the exact time of death and returned to my cot. You would think such a death would be riveting, and it was for the moment. But I had done what my training had called for, performed technically effective CPR and persisted for an appropriate length of time. Intellectually, academically I felt no guilt or inadequacy and I felt little emotion. Fatigue overwhelmed me and I succumbed to sleep as I felt the adrenaline rush subside and my heart rate slow.

"Dr. German, Dr. German, it's 5:30 a.m. . . . Dr. German."

So spoke my human alarm clock, the nurse I had instructed to wake me for rounds.

"O.K. I'm awake."

Who was I kidding? I needed another twelve hours in the sack, but I had twelve hours of work ahead of me. So started another day on the Red Service, and sleep, which I craved for more than food or spousal arousal, eluded me once again.

The work week was grueling; however Saturday was a special treat. Carol and Lynn brought a homemade supper to the hospital. To avoid "Malignant Stan" in the cafeteria, we snuck up to the top floor of the building. We walked onto the flat gravel roof of the hospital. Three weathered folding chairs and an old card table served as our dining room. We wiped off the cardboard table and sat down on the somewhat rickety chairs. When Carol opened our picnic basket, the warm smell of hot dogs cut up into chunks floating in a pot of delicious Boston baked beans, warm homemade brown bread and butter floated from beneath the cloth napkins.

"Daddy, Daddy, look your favorite. Mommy made your favorite meal and I helped, too!"

"Lynn, I'm so proud of you. It smells so good." I glanced at Carol and smiled in appreciation of her efforts. "Thanks."

She looked away as our daughter scrambled into my lap.

Munching a hunk of steaming brown bread with butter melting on top, Lynn curled into my shoulder. This was a traditional Connecticut treat my mom made on Sunday night, and the smells instantly transported me back to being a little boy. I was nostalgic for less stressful times.

Carol took my hand. "Rich, you look tired. Are you okay?"

"Here Daddy, eat your bread." Lynn urged, and then told her mother." My daddy isn't tired."

"I was up most of the night on an emergency aneurysm. Took a nap a few hours ago. I'll be okay."

I looked at Carol. She didn't look convinced.

"I think I'm giving up on the idea of going into heart surgery." I floated that out there waiting for her reaction. When she said nothing, I continued, "I never thought it would be this hard." That certainly was part of it.

"Take your time, Rich. You'll be off the Red Service in two weeks. Right now you're exhausted. Give yourself time." She kissed me on the cheek as she squeezed my hand.

Lynn made a drawing for me and we sang our song, "*California Dreamin'*".

We made a perfect duet.

Time to return to work. I had postponed two new admits in order to eat supper with Carol and Lynn. Sitting on the top of the hospital, 9 stories high of hope and loss, blood and guts, raw emotions and miracle cures handcuffed in a curriculum I was determined to finish, and yet I wanted to be an eagle and take flight across the tree tops below, soaring above the street lights and traffic, out and away toward the west, toward the sun setting in the distance. I remember to this day that ephemeral oasis of peace and comfort overlooking the Genesee River and watching the sun inch down to the horizon.

I had a rare Sunday off. We planned a fall picnic near the Finger Lakes three weeks in advance for that Sunday. The day dawned with pouring rain. The weather was irrelevant—I was not to be deterred from my only damn day off in three months. We will picnic in the rain and LOVE it!

Hunched over the steering wheel, eyes squinting through the torrential downpour thumping on the windshield, I drove through suburban Rochester onto US Rte 56 south to the Finger Lakes. Not surprisingly we were the only car in the parking lot, and the only visitors that day.

Carol and Lynn sat in silence as I exited the car and opened the trunk. Pulling umbrellas, basket and a blanket from the car, I started laughing at the steady downpour soaking my hair and running down my neck into my shirt. I held an umbrella over Carol and Lynn as they piled out of the car. We hiked for twenty minutes carrying our picnic supplies beside the river bank. We slipped in the mud, fell on our butts, and rolled around in wet soil, leaves, and twigs. Standing up, Sasquatch had nothing on us. Laughing, we gave up and retreated to the car to enjoy our picnic even though we were soaking wet. God bless Carol and Lynn for putting up with my Type-A personality.

"Duke, Duke, Duke, Duke of Earl...",
Gene Chandler, 1962

"German, you're helping me on an open heart tomorrow. Brush up on aortic valves." So spoke God.

We started the case at 7:30 a.m. Here was the pecking order: the head of cardiovascular surgery, Dr. Earle, was a very distinguished, silver-haired, trim, tanned, erudite and terse individual who carried a big stick. He was known as "The Duke", as in "Duke of Earl", a song that was popular in the early '60's. He always wore the same wing-tipped shoes, highly polished in a reddish hue, which the Chief Resident, sycophant that he was, tried diligently to emulate; the Chief Resident, "Malignant Stan", or "Stan the Man" on his better days, was "The Duke's" first assistant and stood directly across the OR table from him, on the patient's left side. If "The Duke" got frustrated during the case, he rarely took it out on Stan. Rather, he took it out on the lesser beings—that would be the Junior Resident or me.

"I need better retraction".

"Suction the blood out faster".

"Don't assist me. Just help me".

There were some staple comments that would descend from the God level to my level rather rapidly during moments of stress; the Junior Resident, who was closest to me in hierarchy and therefore somewhat friendly, would nevertheless distance himself from incompetence so as to deflect any possible blame or implication. He and Stan would speak in barely discernible tones during the case to insure the next instrument would be ready and yet not distract "The Duke". He stood to the left of Stan, next to the scrub nurse. Lucky him—she was a babe! Even "The Duke" acknowledged that...

The most expendable, least important, speak-only-if-spoken-to individual in the room, and that, of course, would be me, the silent intern. I was the roving member of the team since I would be directed to different positions around the table as needed: Suction here, retract there.

An anesthesiologist, a float nurse, who would float about the room as needed, the pump tech who maintained the open heart-lung machine or "pump", were the other professionals in the room. Occasionally the cardiologist who had referred the case attended the surgery. He was the one person in the room that I felt superior to, not in knowledge but at least in OR stature—I had gloves on, he didn't (only the surgical team wore gown and gloves). That was my own private little ego boost for the day—an intern had to take whatever he could in strokes.

"The Duke" took the knife and made a long midline incision the entire length of the sternum. Bleeding was controlled, the skin retracted and the glistening cartilaginous sternum was completely split down the middle with an oscillating saw that splattered blood and spicules (tiny fragments) of cartilage over the drapes. Stan the Man inserted a large stainless steel retractor between the split halves of the sternum and to avoid cracking the ribs, he slowly cranked it open. We entered the mediastinum, revealing the beating heart, enclosed in its thick covering, the pericardium. Forceps in hand, "The Duke" and Stan picked up a pinch of the pericardial sac and made a cut between the forceps, taking great care to avoid the phrenic nerve which runs along the pericardial surface. The phrenic nerve innervates the diaphragm and allows for spontaneous respiration. Cut the nerve and the patient can't breathe. That is just one of the many landmines in surgery.

With the pericardium opened and reflected back, the heart surface became fully visible—the dark, red, thick walled muscular ventricles contracting vigorously, the blue-gray thin walled atria with their delicate appendages looking like tiny feet of an embryo contracting just prior to the ventricles, and thick plates of bright yellow fat covering the upper ventricles like a melting glacier.

This incredible organ beats all on its own, 100,000 times a day, 36 million times a year, and two and one-half billion times in a person's life. It pumps 1,500 gallons of blood a day, half a million per year, 35 million in a lifetime—that's enough to fill over 400 swimming pools. And it does so without a switch or a plug. Cut it out of the body and it continues beating devoid of its own blood or oxygen! It is a miraculous organ only the size of your fist.

A large tube was placed into the right atrium to collect deoxygenated blood (blood low in oxygen) returning to the heart and sending it on to the pump. A second tube was placed in the large femoral artery in the groin to receive oxygen rich blood from the pump which then would be dispersed to the entire body, then back again to the right atrium.

The pump had been filled with appropriate cross-matched, compatible blood and was already running. The clamps on the tubes were removed and the pump took over circulating and oxygenating the blood. The heart became motionless by intent, packed in a saline ice slurry and quickly stopped beating. Now came the serious stuff.

The atriae were cut open revealing 3 of the 4 valves crusted and thickened by rheumatic heart disease, caused by rheumatic fever following an untreated strep throat infection 30 years earlier. Back then, Margaret had been a young girl (one consequence of rheumatic fever can be a pathological inflammatory reaction of the heart valves to antibodies produced by the body to neutralize the Streptococcus bacteria). Over time, under the insidious influence of the streptococcal bacteria, the valves progressively deteriorated to the point of non-function, driving the heart to do an incredible amount of work just to get blood out into the body. As the valves worsened, so did the heart efficiency coefficient and the patient grew more and more weary until her tolerance for even minor physical exertion was severely compromised. This led her to seek medical attention, and now all I could see of her was the inside of her motionless heart and those diseased valves that looked like the bulbous nose on W. C. Fields.

The tricuspid, mitral and aortic valves all needed replacement. Each valve had to be excised with Metzenbaum scissors, and then replaced with a prosthetic valve.

Surgery had started at 7:30 a.m. and it was now 1 p.m. The first valve had been inserted and sutured in place. Part way into the second valve a complication occurred. The inside of the heart was tearing where the valve was being sutured, and the valve had to be removed.

Two hours later the second valve was in and I broke scrub to go pee. I re-gowned and gloved and the nurse fed me orange juice through a straw she stuck under my mask. The third valve wasn't going well either. It was now 4 p.m., 8 ½ hours into the surgery, and my back was stinging. Then fatigue set in—such terrible fatigue I had to bite the side of my tongue and pinch my arm with a clamp to try to stay awake. The nurse squeezed a sponge filled with alcohol down the back of my neck and it streamed all the way down to my butt. It sent an electric shock through me that temporarily did the trick.

Then one complication after the other started to happen, like dominoes following the path of least resistance with no way to stop them. The patient had been on pump for over 8 hours—survival for pump time beyond 7 hours drops precipitously for complex physiological reasons.

We were faced with a "no win" situation—take her off pump with an incomplete operation, and she would not survive; persist, and only prolong the inevitable. Two more hours. "The Duke" continued the surgery."

After nearly 12 hours on the table, we had no choice but to take the patient off pump. Her heart could not support her own physiologic needs, her blood pressure sank and her poor, tired, exhausted failing heart gave up. We broke scrub, removed our bloodied gown and gloves and left the OR in silence.

Neither before nor since in all my surgical years have I felt such complete mental or physical exhaustion. A whirlwind of emotions hit me as I laid down on the gurney outside the OR and closed my eyes. I saw her face and heard her voice asking me the night before surgery, "Doctor, will I be OK? Will I make it through surgery?"

I could feel her cold, boney hand in mine as I remembered leaning toward her in an effort to reassure her.

"Margaret, you have the best heart surgeon, the best surgical team and the best technicians. You're going to do just fine. I'll come in to see you after the case is over".

My heart was pounding as I repeated her questions over and over, and felt the somber hand of her death and my fatigue pull me down into a deep sleep.

Part of a doctor's maturation process is to become less and less emotionally self-indulgent and more and more objective. This process carries through all levels of medical education, and for some it's easier than for others. The bottom line is, for maximum efficiency and expertise, which is what we get paid for, emotional involvement must take a back seat to stoicism and performance.

Everyone had his own take on the Red Service as the intern. We were in 100% agreement, however, on the overriding, dominant factor that controlled our lives during that interminable one month rotation—abject fatigue. One night, months later, while rotating on the Plastic Service, an absolute cake walk by comparison, I was finishing up a long day. It was 11:30 p.m. and I walked down the hallway past a patient room. A dim light was on and the patient, a new admit, was giving his health history to the doctor. The doctor was the Red Service intern sitting in the bedside chair sound asleep while the patient happily droned on about his gall bladder, tonsillectomy and appendix. The patient was blissfully unaware his physician was equally unaware of him.

Been there, done that.

I kept on walking down the hallway, out of the hospital and continued my five minute walk home to the university apartments reserved for grad students and medical house staff. It was late September—a definite chill was in the air and I enjoyed the brisk walk home, knowing I had a warm bed waiting rather than a damn cot stuck in the corner of the ICU.

Winter came early that year, and with it the cold air blast off Lake Ontario. Nothing has ever hit me like a Rochester storm—we got a quick 2 foot dump of snow…and shortly thereafter an influx of broken hips from the senior citizens. I was on the Ortho Service then and looking forward to the complexities of repairing bones and reattaching muscles. After a freezing rain, an ice slick often covered streets and sidewalks. It looked as if God had poured gelatin over the entire landscape and it was treacherous for anyone venturing out onto those slippery streets, especially for an elderly person with poor balance with only a worthless cane to support them.

These patients were at a higher risk of forming blood clots in their legs which could break loose and be carried up the large venous pipeline called the vena cava to the right atrium, then into the right ventricle. From here, they could lodge in the lungs, as a pulmonary embolus. Consequently, these patients were placed on prophylactic (preventative) IV heparin, a powerful blood thinner. If the dose is too high, the patient is at risk for internal bleeding. In order to determine the appropriate dose of heparin, which is given every six hours intravenously (q6h IV), the health care practitioner checked the patient's clotting time.

Unfortunately, it is not as simple as putting the patient's blood on a slide and looking at your watch until it clotted. Blood is drawn from the patient and 1 cc placed in each of three test tubes. The technician tilts the first test tube every 30 seconds, allowing the blood to contact the inside surface of the test tube until it shows clotting. Then the second tube is tilted until clotting occurs, and finally the technician tilts the third test tube. The moment clotting occurs in the third tube is the "clotting time", usually in the 5 to 12 minute range. Less than five minutes, more heparin is prescribed. More than 12 minutes, less heparin is given (nowadays the lab determines clotting time in an automated fashion). Note that heparin is given IV q6h, round the clock.

And guess who had to perform the test? Certainly not the lab tech who was too busy in the lab. Oh, no—it fell to the less expensive labor of the intern (remember the pay at 68 cents an hour). At 2 a.m. (or 12 midnight or 4 a.m.), my beeper would go off, I would emerge from my soft bed in the resident dorm (you never took call from home) and walk out into a 2 a.m. Rochester blizzard in my scrubs and across the four lane Crittenden Boulevard—no jacket or coat, just my scrubs, I began emerging from my sleepwalking mode and was now in the warm bowels of the University hospital.

That night, I walked into the patient's room with my blood drawing apparatus. The patient was an irascible, confused elderly woman who took no delight in seeing me standing there, needle and syringe in hand. I applied the rubber tourniquet to her skinny upper arm, much to her displeasure, and a succulent ante cubital vein bulged out. I couldn't miss. She yelled in gibberish phrases as she flailed her arm and drove the needle through the vein resulting in a monster hematoma.

My reaction was anger: at her response, at her need for me to be there in the middle of the night, and finally at the needle for penetrating the vein into the muscle. I was only trying to help her. In a moment I realized we had one thing in common—neither had an appreciation for the other. Taking a deep breath, I resolved my frustrations, called for a nurse to steady her arm, and with some luck managed to hit a good vein and drew blood. Then it was time to begin the laborious chore of tipping one glass tube after the other until the blood in the third tube finally clotted. With that information I adjusted the next dose of IV heparin, stumbled out of the hospital through the snow and back into my warm, cozy dorm bed. Unless, of course, my beeper went off to call me into emergency surgery...another day in the life.

His Royal Highness, the Chair of Surgery

Every member of the surgical program was invited to meet individually with Dr. Robbins. You did not want to see another invitation to meet with him until you had successfully completed the program. A second invitation usually meant you were invited to leave.

World renowned for his pioneering work in vascular surgery, Dr. Robbins, the Chair of Surgery, was known for his brilliant carotid artery surgery. Tall and slender, with a narrow head and narrower eyes pinched above a sharp aquiline nose, his white hair in elegant wings swept back from his balding head, this very British doctor closely resembled an American Eagle. Proud, strong, and lord of all he surveyed, he carried a heavy caduceus, ruled with an iron fist and had the power of life and death over his house staff (residents and interns). Every conceivable diploma and honorary degree covered his office walls. There were also letters of gratitude from former patients who were effusive in their praise for his skill, professionalism and success. [Note: you could screw up on rounds, get angry at a fellow intern or resident, yell at a nurse, or forget to kiss your wife good-night, but you were never to be the source of friction or irritation in any form whatsoever for Dr. Robbins. The penalty was always the same—severed genitalia and being shuffled off to a grade B residency program.]

Most OR's are located in the lower floors of the hospital, but at the University of Rochester's hospital, the OR was on the top floor. When surgery was done for the day, the entire entourage would leave the OR in clean scrubs and white lab coats for rounds—Dr. Robbins, the senior and junior residents and intern. Like ducks in a row, Dr. Robbins led the way and we followed in proper pecking order.

The shortest route to the clinical tower was out of the OR, down the hall, out the exit door and onto the flat roof of the hospital, across the roof to the secret tower door and onto the clinical floor. Although this route saved five minutes of walking, no one else was allowed to take this short-cut under penalty of death; as long as Dr. Robbins led the way, we were part of the privileged few.

One late afternoon while crossing the roof, Dr. Robbins stopped by a small storage shed for tools and equipment. The shed was tiny, about 6 by 8 feet, and the door was ajar. Apparently curious, Dr. Robbins leaned toward the door, cocking his head as if listening for something or someone who would reveal the contents of the shed.

He gently opened the flimsy, plywood door. The tools and equipment had been shoved to one side, in their place were a mattress, sheets and blanket from the OR, incense, candle and a portable transistor radio artfully arranged, converting the out-building into a cozy room.

Standing straight as a Coldwater Guardsman, Dr. Robbins rubbed his chin, his brow furrowing in thought. He turned to face his entourage and in a proper British accent, he declared his diagnosis. "What we have here, gentlemen, is a sex nest. I will assume that this is not the domain of any general surgical house officer as this would definitely be beneath his station. I'm certain that no surgical resident in my program would engage in such a sublime act amongst such mundane surroundings."

Unconsciously, we all straightened up at attention before marching onward behind him the rest of the way.

Dr. Robbins' reputation attracted patients from all over the United States and Europe to have their carotid endarterectomy (cleaning out the plaques from the carotid artery to prevent a stroke). As the body ages, cholesterol and calcium deposits can form on the delicate inner lining of the carotid artery. This is called arteriosclerosis. The arterial wall is composed of three layers—the inner lining is the endothelium and should look like the inside of a straw, smooth and perfect; the middle layer is composed of smooth muscle, or muscularis, which allows the artery to constrict or dilate under orders from the autonomic nervous system (sympathetic to constrict, parasympathetic to relax); and the outer layer is the adventitia, a protective covering for the other two layers while maintaining the integrity of the vessel.

Plaque slowly builds up on the endothelium converting the straw's smooth lining into the inside of a rusty pipe. Plaque tends to form at a bifurcation, a fork in the road, such as the division of the main carotid artery into the internal and external carotid arteries. They carry oxygenated blood into the brain (internal carotid) or into the face and neck regions (external carotid). The laminar flow may become slightly turbulent at the bifurcation, and this irritation over years and years is translated into plaque formation because of genetic and/or biochemical predisposition. The name "carotid" comes from the Greek noun "karotides" meaning arteries of the neck, and "karos" meaning heavy sleep, for good reason: if you press firmly on the carotid on the side of your neck, blood flow to the brain is abruptly interrupted and one promptly "falls asleep", a euphemism for unconsciousness.

Composed of tiny fragments, plaque can break off and be carried rapidly up into the brain, causing a TIA (transient ischemic attack) or a completed stroke. Eighty-five percent of strokes are caused by occlusion of a tiny vessel in the brain from either a plaque fragment or an errant blood clot that has broken away from the left atrium of the heart and is associated with atrial fibrillation, an erratic heart rhythm. The other fifteen percent of strokes are formed by a bursting blood vessel in the brain, called a berry aneurysm since it is shaped like a round berry. TIA is transient, lasting one to five minutes, with complete recovery, but can be a precursor to the real thing, a completed stroke. TIA manifests as either sudden loss or severe reduction of vision in one eye only (amaurosis fugax), slurred speech, or unilateral weakness in an arm or leg. All symptoms are transient since the tiny vessel becomes only partially occluded, and oxygenated blood is able to rescue the brain tissue and eliminate the ischemic insult.

We scrubbed up—Dr. Robbins, the senior resident and I. The patient was an 80 year-old VIP from Canada, with a history of TIA and a carotid angiogram revealing plaque formation in LICA (left internal carotid artery).

The patient was on his back and intubated (breathing tube placed down through his larynx and into the upper main stem bronchus, or breathing tube). His head was turned to the right side, fully exposing his left neck which was completely prepped and draped.

Dr. Robbins made a 3 ½ inch long, slight oblique incision parallel and anterior to the sternocleidomastoid (SCM) muscle (turn your head firmly to the right and feel the big prominent muscle that runs from behind your left ear down to the upper part of the sternum, or breastbone—this is the SCM muscle). The carotid artery lies deep in the neck in treacherous territory: molest or damage the hypoglossal nerve and tongue motor function will be severely impaired; tear the internal jugular vein and you have a potential vascular nightmare; injure or cut the vagus nerve and sacrifice the parasympathetic nerve input to the heart, vessels, stomach and internal organs. There are only two grades for this surgery, A + or F. There is nothing in between.

After giving the patient IV heparin to prevent his blood from clotting during the procedure, Dr. Robbins avoided all these landmines with skill, then surrounded and clamped the carotid artery above and below the plaque. He made a 1-inch linear cut in the carotid artery as it branched into the internal and external carotid arteries, thus exposing the plaque. He deftly dissected this area away from the middle layer of the artery, removing plaque and damaged intima together. My job was to suction blood from the wound, to make no inadvertent movement and remain "invisible". Namely, do no harm, make no waves, speak no thoughts!

With meticulous attention to detail, Dr. Robbins removed all tiny, 1-2mm fragments of loose intima (the delicate, innermost lining of a blood vessel) that would have the potential to break off and fly up into the brain once the vessel was sutured and the clamps removed. Tragically, this is exactly what happened, though we didn't know it at the time.

Once the instruments were removed and the skin closed, the patient was extubated, tube removed from his windpipe, and awakened.

"How do you feel, Mr. Peters?"Dr. Robbins asked.

"Uh, uh, uh, uh, uh, mmmmm."

Mr. Peters responded unintelligibly.

My heart pounded at his reaction.

I felt sweat pool in the palms of my hands within the gloves.

The remnants of my inadequate, rushed breakfast began to back up, as I listened to Dr. Robbins talk to his patient.

"Mr. Peters, please, squeeze my hand." Dr. Robbins gently grasped the patient's right hand.

No squeeze.

"Mr. Peters, try to squeeze my hand."

Still, no squeeze.

"Mr. Peters, squeeze with your left hand."

The resident gently lifted Mr. Peter's left hand. I watched the resident's eyebrows lift as he felt the patient's hand respond.

Good squeeze.

No speech.

No use of his right arm.

He had feeling in his right arm, because in a stroke you lose motor ability, not sensation.

Mr. Peters had had a completed stroke...and he had it on the OR table —an absolute disaster.

Silence engulfed the surgical team.

Nothing was said.

Nothing to say.

Dr. Robbins marched from the OR, the resident and I followed. In proper pecking order, I brought up the rear.

Showtime!

We went to the waiting room to talk with the family.

Dr. Robbins broke our self-imposed silence when he addressed the family. I avoided looking at them, because by then I was familiar with the anxious, fearful expressions on the faces of the interested parties waiting for the news from "God", the super surgeon, Dr. Royal Robbins.

Subdued, professional and soft-spoken, Dr. Robbins addressed the group. "Well, grandfather had a bit of a go during the operation." He paused. "You will notice his speech is a bit garbled". Translation—totally aphasic and unable to speak.

He sighed before continuing, "And he may have some weakness on his right side". Translation—permanently wheelchair bound and unable to use his right arm whatsoever. Since the surgery was on the left carotid artery which feeds the left brain, and since the left brain controls the motor power to the right arm and leg, plus speech, the patient got the worst of both worlds.

My heart was pounding. I prayed for invisibility—that my very existence would be briefly transformed into nothingness. I felt the family's eyes darting from Dr. Robbins to the Senior Resident to me and back to Dr. Robbins. I felt so, so helpless, and perhaps a bit guilty that I had been part, albeit a miniscule part, of the surgical team that had resulted in disaster for both patient and family. I feared the potential wrath of Dr. Robbins for the same reason—that I had been a member of his surgical team and had contributed nothing, absolutely nothing. I was standing on very, very thin ice with the real possibility I would break through into deep, icy submersion.

Although, he gave no indication of anything unusual in the outcome of the procedure, I am certain Dr. Robbins was facing his own demons, this time and every time the unusual and unexpected occurred "on his watch". The Hippocratic Oath states, "First, do no harm".

As the year moved on, my surgical exposure increased. I repaired lacerations in the ER, helped in wound closure in the OR, removed "lumps and bumps" under local anesthesia in the clinic and first assisted in more advanced cases when I rotated through the VA Hospital. The Senior Resident and I were the only ones responsible for surgical cases (i.e. no meddlesome Junior Resident to shoulder me out of the way).

I learned more from this experience than any other, thanks to a considerate, personable and confident Senior Resident. He gave me the opportunity for the greatest technical experience of internship and here I "learned to fly". Away from the paranoia and intimidation of the University hospital, he encouraged me to take responsibility, and clearly enjoyed the teaching process. Yes, I made mistakes, and no, I didn't kill anyone. When I erred, he corrected me with guidance, not reprimand. He was an oasis of encouragement and information, and made me hopeful for my future in surgery.

Often the Senior Resident is more concerned about his "rice bowl" than educating and mentoring his charges, the Junior Residents and Interns. When that happens it robs both sides of the equation of valuable experience.

The year swept by quickly, even though it was what I consider the most grueling and unpleasant year of my training. The prevailing attitude that filtered from the top down, from Chief Resident to intern, was "I suffered, so shall ye suffer." Errors were inevitably made, and the result was humiliation—not the best teaching method. One rapidly became stoic, tough, compulsive and competitive and at times succumbed to anger.

One evening I was grabbing a bite with an ENT resident who had a decent sense of humor.

"Rich, do you know the definition of a New England puritan?" He grinned between bites of a Sloppy Joe sandwich.

I shook my head "no" as I attacked my double cheeseburger loaded with catsup, mustard, mayo and lettuce. As usual, it tasted like a mass of wet chewy mystery meat and dry crunchy cardboard bread. But, I was hungry, and I knew from experience the food will fill the hole in my belly...for a few hours at least.

"It's the haunting fear that someone, somewhere just might be having a good time!" he said with a deep, resounding laugh.

Funny how a joke serves as a catalyst.

The punch line went directly to my heart, as I had not had a good laugh, or truly enjoyed myself for far too long. In fact, the lack of sleep, the pressure, and for the first time in my life I seriously considered the need to escape, to get the hell out of there to maintain my sanity.

My marriage was slowly deteriorating and I couldn't blame it all on internship. Carol and I never raised our voices to each other; we had no "issues" that I was aware of, and there were no tensions, pressures, or conflicts to create a tidal wave of passion. We were best friends, shared everything, including understanding of each other's challenges, and we loved our daughter completely. However, it is possible to love one's child and no longer be "in love" with her parent.

The demands of four years in college, four years of med school and this exacting internship weighed heavily on me, and I knew I would not make it through another five years of surgical residency without a break. I felt like a marathon runner faced with a 26.2 mile race. At the 20 mile point I was fatiguing, my legs were starting to cramp, and my lungs were burning. But only 6.2 miles to go. By mile 24 the sweat was stinging my eyes, my neck muscles were aching and I could not hold my head up. I didn't have the energy to spare on moving my eyes around, so I looked down at the ground, following the road, yard by yard. There, at last, was what I thought to be the finish line, only to be told I had five more years of residency. I needed a break.

It turned out to be a rather dramatic and complete break.

CHAPTER TWENTY FOUR

A PARADIGM SHIFT

"In the depths of winter I finally learned that within me there lay an invincible summer."
Albert Camus, French author

"War" (What Is It Good For),
Edwin Starr, 1970

June 30, 1968 arrived, our last night as interns. We had been tethered to our pagers for twelve months, nearly 24-7, and we went out to the local watering hole for a beer—a very rare treat. We told stories, reminisced about the previous twelve months, and the departure of "Malignant Stan" who was leaving for private surgical practice.

Dave Jones, blond, blue-eyed and the All American Intern, was leaving the next day to be a flight surgeon in the Air Force. "If there is one thing I have learned over the last twelve months it is that I refuse to spend another twelve months here. I'll take Viet Nam over this place any day."

As he stood up to leave, his pager went off. He looked at it as if it was an insignificant part of his attire, and then very deliberately he removed it from his belt, dropped it in the pitcher of beer and walked out.

The rest of us finished the beer and left the pager in the empty pitcher.

Pauper to Prince

The next morning, July 1st, 1968 was my first day as a surgical resident. Suddenly in one day I had gone from being "an incompetent and potentially dangerous intern" to a junior resident. Funny, I didn't feel any different, but now it was my turn to steer an intern away from trouble. Part of the process is cramming so much practical information, hands-on experience, and the "reality" of medicine into a brain limited by lack of sleep and shortage of time to absorb all of it. This creates a lightning fast time warp that spits the intern out, a year older and a century wiser...even though he is unaware of the wiser part....yet.

For now the shoe had shifted to the other foot——no longer the kicked, we became the kicker of the next person below us on the ladder. Resembling "Flounder" from the movie "Animal House", Fred Scales, an intern, had just arrived in Rochester that sunny, humid morning. Fleshy, and out of shape, Fred struggled to keep up with the rest of us as we made rounds on several floors of patients. Of course we were still not allowed in the elevators, so each flight of stairs resulted in his lagging farther behind. Huffing, puffing and sweating we heard him gasp his way into the room at the rear of the entourage already assembled at the bedside of the next patient. Within two weeks he was replaced by another intern. To this day I don't know whether he quit, transferred or just dropped out.

One day another face with another name tag appeared, and life went on.

I remember thinking, "That ain't going to happen to me". From that moment, I ran up the stairs two at a time.

We were too busy, too involved in patient care, and too committed to the immediate task at hand to wonder what had happened to "Flounder". The Hell of internship was a distant memory, and this was a piece of cake by comparison. All you had to do was work hard. You didn't worry about surviving anymore—that was the goal of internship. The prescient words of the admissions secretary five years earlier came back to me in a rush—"If you had the stamina to hitchhike all night in the driving rain, and then go through three interviews, you'll make it through med school."

Stamina and endurance. Two huge assets for what most people consider a strictly intellectual discipline.

As a first year resident, I had the opportunity to choose among several rotations.

Synthetic Surgery for Synthetic Surgeons?

One rotation was plastic surgery, as benign a service as one could find in an otherwise uptight back-East residency program. The East Coast education had the reputation of being all business, no frills, and no bullshit...ever. In contrast, the West Coast's laid back, go with the flow approach to academia had real appeal for this specialty.

This was a "gentleman's service" and I loved it, as much for the relaxed atmosphere as for the rotation itself....except for the burn cases, when plastic became preservation.

One evening two homeless black men, living in an abandoned shack, apparently drank too much cheap wine, then fell asleep and woke up on fire from the candles they burned for light. Tall and thin, these men were admitted while unconscious and never said a word during the length of their stay in the hospital.

Each man suffered third degree burns over 40% to 50% of their torsos and lower extremities from their burning clothing. First degree burn is sunburn, second degree is blister formation to partial thickness burn (involves the epidermis but only part of the dermis), and third degree is full skin thickness burn (involves the entire dermis at the very least) and can extend into deeper tissues of fascia and muscle. The "Rule of Nines" represents percentage of skin surface area of the human body: 18% for each leg, 18% for the entire back, 18% for the entire torso, 9% for each arm, 9% for the head and 1% for the perineum.

Burns are devastating due to pain, multiple organ injuries, massive nutritional demands (patients may require 3,000 or more calories per day), complex and repeated grafting procedures, infection, chronic care, extensive physical therapy and psychological rehabilitation. In the 1970's a significant development in the treatment of burns, was TPN, or total parenteral (as opposed to oral) nutrition was a miraculous IV solution of protein, minerals and high glucose content containing 1 calorie/ml (1000 calories per liter). This enabled patients to sustain their nutritional requirements indefinitely. In the late 1960's this was not available, and nutrition came in the form of an NG (naso-gastric) tube passed into the nostril, down the esophagus and into the stomach. We attached a large funnel to the external end of the tube and poured down a dozen egg whites (pure protein) a day plus peanut butter milk shakes for additional calories. Sounds crude, but it was very effective and life prolonging.

The cost of such global care can be ruinous, and often only the very rich or very poor can afford it. Thermal energy imparted to the skin can lead to absorption of toxins and subsequent damage to the kidneys which attempt to filter out those toxins. This may result in renal failure, a significant and often terminal event in the pre-dialysis days of my training. Inhalation of heat may further damage the delicate mucous lining of the respiratory tree (lungs). The smell of smoke is readily apparent every time the patient exhales. If the damage is severe enough, the bronchial lining will slough and be expelled with a bloody cough. This invariably results in an irreversible downhill course to disaster. These patients require emergent tracheostomy, respirator dependence and high concentration of oxygen which over prolonged periods can be toxic itself. Mortality in such cases is very high, and survival the distinct exception.

Skin grafting, a surgical procedure usually performed under general anesthesia for patient comfort and to reduce operating time, requires preparation of two distinct areas: the burn (recipient) site and the graft (donor) site. The recipient site must first be meticulously debrided of dead tissue, often on several separate occasions to insure a rich, vascular bed capable of supporting and nourishing a free skin graft. The double edged sword is that the thicker the graft the better the coverage and cosmetic result, but the greater the chance of graft failure due to greater vascular demand. A very thin graft will almost certainly "take" but doesn't look as nice or provide the same degree of surface protection. The accepted compromise is a graft mid-way between, about sixteen thousandths of an inch thick. At this thickness, not only will the recipient site get good coverage and heal readily, but the donor site will also fully regenerate and be a source for a repeat donor grafting if those patients who have extensive burn and limited donor site availability need it.

Our team had taken the two burn patients to the OR on multiple occasions for debridement and removal of dead and necrotic burn tissue in order to achieve a suitable bed for grafting. We first prepared the previously debrided burn site by applying moderate abrasion with a saline soaked sponge to stimulate bleeding and remove any residual debris. We then used a CO_2 pressure driven Brown dermatome with a high speed oscillating blade to remove donor skin from the patient's back for grafting onto the extremities. The skin was covered with sterile mineral oil to reduce friction. As the blade sliced into the dermis, the dermatome was slowly advanced with modest downward pressure. The graft peeled away from the blade like a thin slice of deli meat (16/1000 of an inch thick), leaving a path of fresh bleeding in its wake. The donor site was covered with Vaseline impregnated gauze and a dry pressure dressing for control of bleeding.

The free, partial thickness graft was placed over the clean burn site and secured with similar dressings. Occasionally a hand stapler was used to anchor the edges of the graft to the adjacent skin. Every effort was made to prevent bleeding or oozing deep into the graft, since this would lift the graft away from its vascular bed, denying nourishment and resulting in graft failure. The firm application of a dressing was not left to the intern; rather, the primary surgeon gave his stamp of approval to this critically important and final step of the procedure.

In spite of weeks of care, debridement, grafting, antibiotics, nutritional and pulmonary support, both patients eventually succumbed to sepsis and organ failure. I will never forget those two friends, lying side by side in the ICU, struggling independently to survive, showing courage, stoicism and camaraderie until they were separated by death, first one and then the other two days later. A tough life and a cruel ending.

August: ER...

As the emergency room surgical resident, I was called for the big stuff—stab wounds, major trauma, acute abdominal surgery, etc. The minor stuff—lacerations, small burns, foreign bodies were left to the intern (me a year ago).

One evening I was discussing a case with a couple of nurses over jet black coffee and stale chocolate cake. I was feeling almost confident when the piercing scream of a siren descended into the ER receiving area.

"Doc, there's a lady in the ambulance... she's about to deliver. Quick! We need you right away!" The EMT's voice vibrated on the edge of panic as he bounced in place in front of me.

My immediate thought was, "Call for a doctor, a REAL doctor, OB-type." As the young maid Prissy said in *"Gone With the Wind"*, "I don't know nothin' 'bout birthin' babies."

No such luck.

The OB resident was doing a C-section, which left me. I followed the EMT as we both ran into the parking lot. The back doors of the ambulance were wide open, perfectly framing a very large black woman lying with her legs spread to reveal her baby's head emerging.

Falling forward, I immediately placed my hand

against the baby's head to slow delivery down and prevent dangerous decompression which can occur if the baby emerges too precipitously from the birth canal. At least I had remembered something from my OB rotation as a fourth year med student.

"Don't push, don't push," was that my voice? It sounded too high for my voice. "T- Take it slowly, ok, er ma'am?"

Suddenly Mom coughed and out came the baby (No. 5 for Mom) with very little help from me. I applied two Kelly clamps, divided the cord and handed the baby girl off to the nurse. I never got so much credit for so little work in my professional career.

It didn't surprise me when Carol chose not to accompany Lynn and me on those few outings we squeezed in between my hospital requirements. It didn't disappoint me either. That should have been a sign...

But boy, did we have fun on the weekends. I was now making $400 a month as a resident but things were still tight so I started a moonlighting gig. I was the field physician for the high school football games—two every Saturday for $35 a game. I took Lynn with me and she would run up and down the sidelines with the cheerleaders. At half time we ate hot dogs and a coke, sitting on the grass like I was a real dad. These were precious moments and about the best memories I have of my six years in Rochester. Winds of change were in the air.

October Rain...

Three months into my residency Carol and I separated. This was a carefully guarded secret as I was ashamed of my marital failure. I told absolutely no one—not my closest friends, parents or my sister. Lynn was now six and a beautiful little girl. She was so used to me being in the hospital most of the time that it wasn't anything out of the ordinary.

Our marriage died like many patients, a rattle, a sigh, and then nothing. What had begun as a schooner on the open ocean of opportunity, driven by a fair wind and following seas, had becalmed. Not even a breeze for momentum. There were no broadsides from enemy ships, no mutinies aboard, simply a lack of air moving us forward. So, rather than scuttle the ship, we agreed to disembark.

Once we agreed on this course of action, I had to find a place to live. Fortunately, there was always a place to stay in the house staff dorm to tide me over until I found a room for rent. A 3 by 5 hand written card was tacked on the announcement board advertising a room for rent only two miles from the hospital. Carol kept the car, and I used an old bicycle a former resident had given me. In October, this worked fine, but the upcoming Rochester winter was a challenge.

The house was an old, wood two-story place with a pitched roof in a very modest part of town.

The owner of the house, Jack Hardy, was a man who lived alone and was looking for some extra income. He was about 40 years old and very heavy, around 250 pounds on a 5 foot 8 frame. Since the price was right, and there did not appear to be anything else available, I pushed away the uneasy feelings I had the first time we shook hands. His hand was fleshy, which was expected, but his grip was too tight..almost aggressive, as if he was trying to prove something.

His demeanor was a bit unusual, almost flirtatious. He looked at me in a weird way, a beguiling way, a way that made me very uncomfortable.

After introductions, the next thing out of his mouth was "No girlfriends allowed."

Since I had not brought up the subject because I had no girlfriend, his comment seemed odd to me. Anyway, my late night work schedule meant I wouldn't be around much, so our interaction would be minimal. A small price to pay for cheap rent.

For the first few days, either coming or going, I never saw my landlord. Then for several days in a row, he seemed to be up late waiting for me. He tried to engage me in conversation, but I politely begged off telling him that sleep was all I wanted and went into my room.

Those nights I fell asleep almost prior to my head hitting my pillow and slept soundly until the alarm went off—-except once or twice when I awoke for no apparent reason. No lights, no sudden loud noises, just my eyes snapping open and looking around as if someone had popped a balloon behind my head. Lying there in the silence, I wondered what it was that had disturbed my sleep and I heard the door knob turn. My door was locked from the inside, so whoever was trying to enter my room was not able to do so, but his efforts at not being detected were not successful.

Shrugging, I yanked the blankets up over my shoulder and rolled over falling immediately back to a deep sleep. . This happened two more times, and I realized the first time was no accident, so I made up my mind to say something to my landlord the next time I saw him.

Shaving, I sensed rather than saw him walk into the tiny bathroom we shared. He stood nude with just a towel over his shoulder and a smile on his round face. This was not a locker room, we were not friends, and real men didn't do things like that. Ok, so now I have to lock the bathroom as well as my bedroom door when I'm inside...

Days turned into weeks and nothing else unusual occurred so I forgot the earlier instances, and dismissed them as inconsequential.

One night I returned home early, and he asked me if I wanted a beer. It had been quite a while between beers, so I accepted and we moved into his living room. Elsewhere in the world, the Viet Nam war was raging, the political scene was alive with protest, and the cultural scene was full of sex, drugs and rock 'n roll. It wasn't hard to find something to discuss in those troubled times.

Careful not to venture into anything too controversial, we talked casually about the neighborhood changes, the hospital, and eventually our conversation wandered into local politics, one of his favorite subjects.

To make a point he placed his hand on my knee.

HELLO! What the hell is this all about?!

"Jack, I don't know if I'm misinterpreting signals, but I feel you are coming on to me. Am I right?"

"Yes, I'm homosexual," he said softly. "You're an attractive man."

Too stunned to speak, my mouth fell open.

"The thought has entered my mind," he continued.

"Well, Jack, put it out of your mind!" I said, recovering. "I'm not homosexual." "End of story," I said, as I stood up to leave the room.

He appeared disappointed but seemed to accept my statement.

To make sure, I always arrived late at night, long after he was asleep.

Or so I thought.

It was a cold, snowy February night. I parked my bicycle on the front porch and quietly made my way up the creaky wood stairs. After I brushed my teeth in dark silence, I went to bed. Dogged tired from a long shift, I fell asleep quickly. Again, something strange woke me up, pulling me from the depths of sound sleep, slowly at first; and then a blast of adrenaline shot electric impulses up my spine.

I felt massive weight on the side of my bed. There he was all naked 250 pounds sitting on the side of my bed as he touched himself. A dim ceiling light bulb in the hallway offered minimal visibility, but his facial expression and intention were unmistakable.

"I want you in the worst way," his whisper was filled with saliva.

Horrified doesn't begin to explain my feelings at that moment. My heart was pounding. I was scared shitless. Afraid he'd jump me and I'd have to fight my way out. I had to put a stop to his fantasies, STAT!

"Look. Leave me ALONE! We've been over this before. PLEASE just leave me ALONE NOW!

He grumbled, stood up and left my room. I watched him until I saw my door closing behind his big fat hairy ass. My heart rate was close to 130. Lying in bed for what seemed like hours, I strained to hear the creak of a floor board, the whisper of the door knob, the flick of a light switch in the hall. When I was sure he was asleep, I pulled on my pants, sweater, jacket, socks and boots, packed up all my belongings in a duffle bag and crept down the stairs and out into the bitter cold blizzard. Strapping my bag to the back of the bike, I pedaled off into the storm. My watch said 3:00 A.M. The deserted neighborhood road had not been recently plowed, so the scene was eerily quiet as the snow fell nearly horizontal against the dim streetlight.

I was disgusted. I shook my head side to side to keep the snowflakes out of my eyes. I yelled out loud, the cold air turning my breath into visible bursts of anger. "Richard, how the hell did you get yourself into this terrible position?!" Six years in this God-awful city. Separated from your wife and nearly raped. And surgery in four hours. "Damn you!—Get your shit together!" Every word froze the air in front of me, visible bursts of anger, self-loathing, and shame.

This was the nadir. I was down, really down, but I was far from out. I pedaled my way to the hospital through the falling snow; each down stroke of the pedal renewed my momentum toward getting out of the shit hole I was in. I gained strength knowing that a paradigm shift was at hand. For just a moment, a very brief moment, time cracked open for me and I saw a vision of my future that seemed immutable, inevitable and most of all, liberating.

"We Gotta Get Out of This Place",
Eric Burdon and The Animals (1965)

I saw a means to find my strength, and with it a new direction and meaning for my life. I knew then and there I would stop this downward spiral. A new reality came over me in a rush. I would join the Navy as a surgeon, even if it meant Viet Nam. The decision made, I coasted the rest of the way to the hospital.

After two hours of sleep, loaded up on caffeine, I walked into the OR and scrubbed up. No one in that room had any idea what I had just been through.

The nurse handed me the knife.

After a week in the resident dorm I found a room to rent, this time from an 82 year-old lady who loved the idea of leaving my big boots inside the porch door "to scare off any robbers". She became my surrogate grandmother, making cookies for me to eat when I arrived home late. Often she stayed up watching television at nearly full volume. So as not to startle her I would bang my feet on the floor when I got home, take off my boots and shout "Hi, Mrs. Winters" in a loud voice. As I walked into the T.V. room she would suddenly jerk her arms up and say, "Oh! You gave me such a start!" From then on I would flick the light switch to alert her—no more "starts".

I drove to Buffalo for my Navy physical. All the things I routinely did to my patients now were done to me. Standing naked in line with eight other guys bent over with butts at the ready was not exactly a privacy moment. Welcome Aboard!

After nearly six years in Rochester, I had three months to go in my residency. My Navy commission as a Lieutenant was confirmed, and my orders to Da Nang indicated in bold letters.

The thought flashed through my mind—on July 1st, 1969 I would not morph into a second year resident in surgery. I would instead be a full Lieutenant in the Navy, wearing a khaki uniform and two silver bars on my shoulder. This was the paradigm shift I had been waiting for and I could feel it well up inside me like a tsunami.

Thirteen years of study, tests, competition, long hours, fatigue and personal and financial strain seemed to melt away and I no longer felt the pressure to perform. What a sense of liberation! The gnawing fear of failing, so prevalent among med students and the driving force to over-achieve, drifted away in an amorphous cloud.

The wind had shifted...

My energy seemed limitless. I ran across campus, played touch football like a maniac and powered through difficult surgical cases with room to spare. I was more than happy to help a fellow med student and his wife move into their new digs off campus; an all-day affair of lifting dead-weight furniture, carrying overstuffed boxes and dragging a second-hand fridge across the floor. Then came time for pizza and beer. But something unusual happened, and rather suddenly. Not only was I totally exhausted, but I had no appetite. I slumped down onto their monster couch and closed my eyes.

"Hey, Rich. Eat this. You'll feel better."

My host handed me a thick juicy piece of hamburger pizza overflowing with mozzarella cheese and tomato. What should have made me hungry turned my stomach.

"I think I'm going to throw up".

"Rich, you don't look so good".

He helped me off the couch and I made it to the bathroom—barely. I thought I was going to faint. I knelt on the floor and rested my head on the toilet seat. A wave of nausea rushed over me and then subsided.

I thought to myself "What in the hell is the matter with me?" I drooled saliva into the toilet then slowly stood up to pee. Holy shit! My urine was the color of dark beer. I immediately looked into the mirror and I was icteric—

the whites of my eyes were bright yellow. Oh Christ, Richard, you've got hepatitis!

Next stop—the hospital.

After checking me in, the ER staff paged the assistant professor of medicine to consult. At 5' 9" tall, pudgy and balding, with a soft reassuring approach, Dr. Pomeroy examined me carefully. I winced when he pressed his fingers just below my right costal margin over the liver edge.

Then he gave me the velvet harpoon—a rectal exam that belied his gentle demeanor.

A flood of nausea swept over me.

"We're going to run some tests, Richard. I'll be back."

"What are you thinking, Dr. Pomeroy?"

"I think you have hepatitis."

In came the lab tech to draw my blood. He put the rubber tourniquet on my left upper arm and my antecubital vein bulged out.

"You've got nice veins, Doc."

"Yeah, thanks." What I meant was "Don't miss!"

I looked away as he inserted a 21-gauge needle through my skin and into the vein. I had done this procedure a thousand times and knew exactly what it looked like. Now I knew what it exactly felt like (I had already learned the trick of stretching out my patient's skin with my left thumb before inserting the needle—it's painless!).

I closed my eyes, feeling vulnerable and mortal, no longer the young lion that I had been just yesterday. All through med school every student feared having one horrible disease after the other as we studied our way from the beginning to the end of that intimidating big, red pathology book by Robbins. A left-sided headache meant an incurable astrocytoma; knee pain must be a potentially fatal osteosarcoma; fleeting chest pain confirmed angina; ringing in the ears certainly pointed to the dreaded acoustic neuroma; and constipation had to be due to a malignant apple-core lesion of the descending colon.

Pathology course meant paranoia, even among supposedly objective, intelligent, healthy med students. Now I was the one lying on the gurney in the ER, contemplating my mortality at age 28. I recognized that the signs and symptoms of nausea, fatigue, tender liver edge, bilirubinuria (bile in the urine) and jaundice damn near confirmed hepatitis, a potentially fatal disease with no cure and only a gamma globulin shot for palliation (hepatitis vaccine is now preventative).

My imagination raced downhill—I pictured myself rapidly progressing from a state of deep jaundice to obtundation, then slipping into coma and death, ending up on a slab in the morgue with Dr. Orbison, our pathology professor, picking up the red-handled autopsy knife and cutting deep into my chest with the standard Y-shaped incision, extending down the midline from my xyphoid process to my pubic bone.

"Richard, you have Hepatitis B".

Dr. Pomeroy was gently touching my right shoulder which jolted me out of my perverted, morbid thoughts and back into reality. I thought to myself, "How in the hell did I get THIS?" Hepatitis B is a contact disease.

Then it hit me—I must have contracted it from a patient the Chief Resident and I performed surgery on over a month ago, and had stuck myself with a round suture needle while closing the abdomen. He turned out to have had Hepatitis B, but I was off the service by then and had not been informed until two weeks post-op.

I hadn't given it much thought. How easily that simple needle stick converted me from a state of complete health to someone with life threatening disease.

I was in the hospital for ten days and each day I grew sicker and more jaundiced. My bilirubin level went from 2.2 mg/dl (normal range is .1 to 1.2 mg/dl) to 10.7 mg/dl and I was yellow as a canary. My urine grew darker, my nausea overwhelming and the only position of comfort was lying on my left side. This position seemed to alleviate the sick feeling of my stomach pressing against my abdomen.

The IV's caloric content was inadequate to meet my caloric needs, and I dropped twelve pounds in ten days, from 183 to 171. I monitored my illness by the color of my urine. Finally, my pee turned from Guinness stout to ale to light beer, and I knew I would make it. "Physician heal thyself" was never more true and I thanked God for the gift of health once again. My body had spontaneously overcome the inflammatory insult temporarily imposed by the Hepatitis B virus by developing the necessary anti-viral antibodies that defeated and eliminated the virus in its tracks, never to rear its ugly head again. This left me immune for life, a type of "internal vaccination".

I was discharged from the hospital and returned to my rented room to recuperate. Mrs. Winters nursed me back to the living on chicken broth and Lipton's tea until my nausea dissipated and my appetite improved. I had missed the entire month of April and could never again donate blood, which had been a source of income for me.

Again, by the grace of God, I did not become a carrier of Hepatitis B antigen, a condition associated with hepatocellular carcinoma (fatal liver cancer). I returned to the hospital as a productive surgical resident, determined to finish my last two months in good status. I was equally determined to vacate Rochester forever and I never divulged my bout with hepatitis to the U.S. Department of the Navy. Neither rain, nor sleet, nor hepatitis, nor Da Nang, would deter me from my personal mission to escape that geographic and psychological ice bowl.

It was now May, with one month left in my first year residency, one month left in my six year training in Rochester, one month left at slave wages and back-East attitude.

I had done my share of surgery, mostly as first assistant, some as primary surgeon. One of my surgical professors had told us he could teach most of the necessary surgical techniques to a resident in 6 months. Teaching is one thing, absorbing the myriad of techniques and the ability to perform under significant stress with maximum efficiency is quite a different matter. The professor's point was that knowledge and judgment are the more difficult assets to acquire for global surgical proficiency.

However, I saw many a senior resident, ready to exit the protection of a training program and enter private practice, with technical skills of varying degrees, some even below par. For the most part, with a few glaring exceptions, those individuals, in time, did master the learning curve. For those exceptions, all the repetition in the world led to no improvement—they were technically inept and, after all, practicing the same technique and expecting different results is a formula for failure.

Those surgeons (I had only known two in 30 years) struggled mightily in private practice, and were beset with a host of surgical complications, had suffered multiple malpractice lawsuits, facing the unkind scrutiny of peer review and ending up with no referrals and no practice. They would have done far better in non-technically demanding fields, i.e. pathology, non-invasive radiology, oncology, family practice, internal medicine or psychiatry. However, asking a man who dreams of surgery to become a psychiatrist (opposite extremes) is like asking a tiger to shed his stripes and become a cow (no offense meant to psychiatrists). To assuage any hurt feelings, the joke is as follows: A surgeon and psychiatrist are talking while the elevator opens. As the doors start to close, the psychiatrist puts his hand in and the surgeon puts his head in (in order to protect his hands at all cost!).

Mrs. Winters was sad to see me go and sent me off with a bag of cookies she had baked. My exit from the University hospital was quiet and anti-climatic. A new set of house staff was arriving and I was leaving for the Navy.

It was 9 AM July 1st, 1969.

We had sent Lynn to Carol's parents near Boston a week earlier. All of our worldly belongings fit into the back seat and trunk of our old Ford, and Carol and I headed out in an uncomfortable silence. It was a hot, humid cloudy day when a lightning bolt blasted a high voltage tower along the turnpike, sending showers of yellow sparks in all directions. Yeah, this was my paradigm shift, and nature was announcing it in a big way.

CHAPTER TWENTY FIVE

"ANCHORS AWEIGH!"

*"Whether we think we can or we can't,
either way we are right."*
Henry Ford, Founder of Ford Motor Co.

"I Like It Like That",
Smokey Robinson, 1964

7 PM July 1st 1969. Tired from the long drive, we pulled into my in-laws' driveway in Taunton, Mass. Lynn dashed from the house to greet us with shrieks of joy. Carol's parents were civil, a testament to the New England stoicism considered the only acceptable behavior in awkward moments. My departure for war was hardly a scene out of "From Here to Eternity" or "Casablanca": no longing, no apparent sadness—simply another leave taken among friends and family.

The next day, July the 2nd, Carol drove me to the Newport, Rhode Island Naval Base one hour away and dropped me off. We were a class of about 30 docs and most of us had been given the rank of Lieutenant. Those with full training came in as Lt. Commanders. All of us were given two weeks of indoctrination: "guns and boats", plus Navy traditions and protocol for good measure. On that first day, all 30 of us sat in a small classroom. We were all strangers, having trained in medical programs from all over the Northeastern section of the country, and lounged in our casual clothes of many colors. Not for long. That afternoon we kissed goodbye to individual wear, and purchased our Navy tans (for work), Service Dress Blues (winter) and whites (Service Dress, and Tropical Longs (for summer), replete with shoulder boards, covers (caps) and shoes. As a Lieutenant, I wore two silver bars on each collar of my tan shirt, and attractive black shoulder boards with two separate gold stripes on my Service Dress Khaki jacket. Shoes were meant to be clean, more of a problem in the summer (white shoes), but docs were never forced to spit shine their blacks. As a group, docs were never held to the same rigid Navy standard as the other officers, each of whom had had to endure OCS (Officer Candidate School) training, and then come up through the ranks: Ensign, Lieutenant Junior Grade, Lieutenant, often four to six years in the process. The rules of saluting dictated the officer of junior rank to initiate the salute, hold it until the officer of more senior rank returned the salute, and then complete the salute. Not a big deal, but some docs were so out of touch that they would initiate a salute to a junior officer or even a non-com, and cause a stir. Even worse was not initiating a salute to a senior officer, a high insult and worthy of disciplinary action which one rebellious doc discovered. He was immediately placed on report, and restricted to his quarters for the weekend, and that was the first weekend in July in Newport, Rhode Island. Navy attitude showed no discrimination geographically. Whether East Coast, West Coast, on the high seas or ashore, Navy protocol demanded the same degree of discipline and respect, regardless. I enjoyed that regimentation; it gave me a secure feeling. I was two days' fresh out of residency and facing my first year in the Navy with an overseas deployment. After that, I wondered where my second year assignment would be. It was totally out of my control, of course, but I couldn't help fantasize and pray that someday I would end up in California.

Originally, my orders were to Da Nang and the major Navy installation that provided surgical care to the wounded ("to the dead and not yet dead" as one anti-war doc sarcastically described it). I was not particularly upset about this assignment. I would be exposed to tremendous trauma and word had it that DaNang was a relatively safe place to be. After a week of rather boring classes on "guns and boats", I was walking the corridor to mess hall and a fellow doc rang out, "Hey, German, go check the assignment sheet in the OD's office—you've been transferred to the 6th Fleet, you lucky dog!" In disbelief I ran down the names in alphabetical order until I reached the "G's": German, R.H., LT.—reassigned to the 6th Fleet. Ship—USS Albany CG-10. Wow! I was going to be the ship's doc aboard a newly commissioned guided missile cruiser headed for the Mediterranean! I couldn't believe it. I thanked my guardian angel and went to the Mess Hall for lunch.

I spent the last day at my in-laws so Lynn and I could have some time together, walking in the apple orchard and talking about fun times. Then it was time to leave. I put on my Service Dress Khaki uniform, said my goodbyes and turned around to blow a final kiss to Lynn. She stood there on the porch, straight as can be, and snapped a smart salute – it still gives me a lump in my throat, not unlike the feeling of watching John John's farewell salute in 1963 to his fallen father, President John F. Kennedy.

I flew to Florida and met my ship in Mayport. What a feeling, walking up to this monstrous 673 foot-long, 180 foot-tall, 19,000 ton all-gray Navy cruiser, bristling with missiles and her pennants whipping in the wind.

"Lieutenant German, reporting. Request permission to come aboard."

"Permission granted, Lieutenant."

A salute to the flag, a salute to the quarter deck and I felt the steel deck beneath my feet. This floating warship would be my home for the next twelve months.

After one week in port, we departed for the U.S. Navy base on the southeastern tip of Cuba (Guantanamo Bay, affectionately known as GITMO). There the ship would conduct naval war exercises, known as an Operational Readiness Inspection (ORI). Occasionally a bloated body, a Cuban shot trying to escape his homeland, floated by our ship. After two weeks at GITMO, and as part of our underway training, we sailed 100 miles off Cuba to test our TALOS missiles against remote controlled aircraft targets known as drones. It was a beautiful summer day and our ship cut through the ocean at about 10 knots. Twelve of us, all officers, were allowed on the very top deck of the ship, 180 feet up. The feeling was absolutely exhilarating, standing in our white uniforms and feeling the wind in our faces, almost as if we had control of the ship and were guiding it due south.

The sun was high in the sky above our heads, and no land, ship or human was in sight. A hydraulic sled guided the 16 foot long, blue and white TALOS missile onto the launcher, its four stabilizing fins at the ready.

The Weapons Officer's voice announced over the ship's loudspeaker.

"Bogie inbound, range 110 miles, bearing 90 degrees. Standby to fire missile:... 4 – 3 – 2 – 1... missile away."

With that the TALOS missile exploded off the launcher with an incredible, piercing blast, the 10 foot long flame scorching the steel deck as it attained Mach 1 in seconds and disappeared as it bore down on the drone somewhere in the distance.

"Missile on course... One minute ten to impact....Missile on course...Thirty-two seconds to impact..Twelve seconds to impact."

Silence.

Followed by more silence.

We stared at the horizon expecting to see a distant flash. Then a small black speck appeared. The speck was moving rapidly toward us and we suddenly realized it was the drone, headed straight toward us.

Propelled by instinct, we dropped to the deck.

The fully intact, totally untouched, rapidly-moving drone passed no more than sixty feet directly overhead the ship, before silently disappearing to the west. Somewhere far to the east the TALOS missile had run out of fuel and entered a watery grave.

So much for weapons' accuracy, circa 1969.

We returned to GITMO for a final week prior to departure for the Med. There was limited activity during downtime so a fellow officer and I went sailing for the day. The Navy had several 26 foot sailboats available to all personnel, and required very little proof of one's nautical ability. My boyhood days spent in Long Island Sound off the Connecticut shore had taught me how to sail, if not to navigate. Hell, there was always a very large, long island to one side or the other of my boat...there was nothing to worry about.

One of my fellow officers trusted me based on my assurance of growing up with sail boats every summer. While my nautical ability had not deserted me, the problem was my lack of attention to our geographic location. After two hours of sailing, we sailed within a half mile of shore. We slowly looked up the hillside until our eyes cast upon a conning tower and machine gun aimed our way. Surprise! Surprise! This was not a welcoming committee from the United States Navy. Instead we had crossed into Cuban waters, and their military had apparently taken offense! Hearts pounding, we came about, and headed back out to sea. Swearing an oath of secrecy, we sailed back to our base.

What a change the Navy was from my former existence. People saluted me. I had a light work load and was pulling in $1,000 a month. Half of it went back to Carol, leaving me with $500 a month and nowhere to spend it. It was winter in Rochester, and I remembered the feet of snow, the harsh bone-chilling winds, the icy unforgiving roads, and the pressure, the competition, the intense survival mode of most of the time I had spent there. Winter is "high season" in the Caribbean, with tropical temperatures and mellow weather. We were headed to Europe, the Mediterranean, and the 6th Fleet, a piece of cake. I had my eye on a Triumph TR-6.

In order to get to Europe, however, we had to cross the Atlantic in February. We hit a whale of a storm—25 foot seas with 19,000 tons of steel ship pitching up and then crashing down bow first into the sea. Green water sucked deeply over the gunwales followed by an explosion of white foam as the entire ship shuttered, straining to free itself and pitch up again. No one was allowed out on deck, since the ship had been rigged for heavy weather due to the high sea state. Lifeline stanchions had been rigged inboard of the normal lines so sailors would have a safe hand hold while topside on the forecastle.

I ventured up the interior ladder to the enclosed Admiral's Flag Bridge, one level below the Captain's bridge. This location provided the best view of the sea's assault on our ship.

The Admiral's bridge was rarely used, but was the exclusive domain for the Admiral and his staff. On this occasion, it was completely empty—a curve of thick bullet-proof glass and several swivel chairs bolted to the deck. To get a bird's eye view of the drama, I sat in the Admiral's chair, dead center of the curve and the best view in the house. For five minutes, strapped in the chair, the ship and I pitched and churned in unison, sea spray blasting up 160 feet to cover the windows. I was so mesmerized by the power and force of nature that I was unaware that the Admiral and staff had entered and were standing behind me.

"And I thought I was the only Admiral aboard."

I whipped around in the chair, tethered by the lap belt, to see a slight smile on the face of Admiral Bennett, surrounded by his staff of four, all wearing the same steely-eyed, frozen stare.

"And indeed you are, Sir," I replied, unbuckling my strap and standing at stiff attention (hard to do with the deck heaving and pitching). With a wink he said, "Be sure to take good care of me when I come down for my annual exam next week."

Translation—be gentle, doctor, and "...do no harm...".

We were being hurled by a following sea. That meant the waves hit the stern of the ship first, sending the bow down towards the water, then traveling through the length of the ship forcing the bow upwards, which then came crashing down with the next monster wave. Worse, it was a quartering sea, one that hit the port aft end of the ship and rolled it to starboard while pitching the bow down. The motion had become so bad that we had to strap ourselves into our bunks. What a great combination—seasick and unable to sleep. And everyone, including the good doctor, got seasick except for the "old salts" that could take anything and had seen everything. Thank God for Dramamine and Saltine crackers!

The storm subsided somewhat as we traveled east toward Europe. However, we were still in a ten-to-fifteen-foot following seas with the ship pitching and rolling. I was called to sick bay to see the ship's Navigation Officer who had a speck of dirt imbedded in the cornea of his right eye.

This was going to be fun, trying to remove a foreign body from the cornea with a #18 gauge needle on a moving target—namely his eye. We strapped the Navigator on the table and immobilized his head. I sat next to him on a stool and had my right forearm taped to his chest so the ship, the Navigator and my right forearm all moved in unison. I placed the heel of my hand on his chin, numbed his eye with Pontocaine drops and told him not to worry. I was the one worrying….more than enough for both of us.

I slowly drew the needle closer to his eye, compensating for the ship's movement and gingerly approached the cornea. I waited for the ship to crest and in that instant flicked off the piece of dirt with the sharp point of the needle.

"Thanks, Doc," a blink, a smile and off he went like it was nothing at all.

What if I had missed? I didn't want to think about it.

We arrived in Gibraltar, Spain in March and spent the next three months cruising the Med. We spent one week in Gaeta, Italy, home of the 6th Fleet and then left for four weeks of sea duty.

I had a lot of down time and not much to do surgically, so I set up a tattoo removal clinic for those sailors who had long since broken up with "Sally" and found a new love to tattoo on their arms. After a few removals, my plastic surgery skills were honed, and I was ready to use my most sought-after talent: circumcisions!

"Hey, Doc, can you have me ready to go in four weeks?"

Every time we left port, I would have a new batch of sailors lined up for their "trim job". Word got around that sex was better for the circumcised. All they cared about was being functional once we pulled into port.

Four weeks later we pulled into Barcelona. The tie lines were ropes the size of a man's thigh, and had three-foot diameter metal cones attached to them half way between the dock and the ship, to prevent rats from climbing up the rope and coming aboard. At the bottom of the ramp I had set up a large sign that had the face of a beautiful Spanish woman with the inscription, "Watch out, sailor, she may have it", a warning against gonorrhea. Imagine, 1200 men, out to sea for four weeks, streaming off the ship in droves, committed to completely ignoring my warnings. Most indeed were very successful and someone wrote in lipstick on my carefully constructed sign, "If she's got it, Doc, we want it!"

And yes, they got it.

Thank God for penicillin.

The sailors' curfew, "Cinderella Liberty", required them to be at the quarter deck by midnight. The totally inebriated ones, supported by their slightly less inebriated buddies, half saluted the flag and officer of the deck and came aboard to sleep it off.

At 0200 hrs. I was called from my bunk to attend a still-drunken sailor who had tried to secretly leave the ship via the mooring lines. He was prevented further progress by the rat guard and was clinging to the rope, singing some unintelligible song about "my beautiful Maria" when he fell straight down 30 feet into the water. By some miracle he had missed the pylons, but he did not miss Captain's Mast the next day, and was not allowed ashore for the rest of the tour.

The Captain has supreme and unchallenged power aboard his ship and his decisions are final and written in stone. Democracy does not apply aboard ship.

On our final night in Barcelona, the Admiral hosted a posh party for officers and political guests on the second floor of a luxurious hotel. It was like something out of the movie, "Officer and Gentleman". All the officers were in their starched Service Dress White uniforms, polished brass and buffed white shoes. I felt privileged and very protected by this special fraternity. It was such a far cry from the competitive dog-eat-dog academia that I had been used to for thirteen years. It was seductive, and so were the cocktails and hors d' oeuvres. But a few of us wanted some local action so we left the party, took a cab, and went to see some authentic flamenco dancing while drinking real Sangria. No beeper, no late night surgery, no abject fatigue. Oh yeah!

At 0300 hrs. We ran out of steam and returned to the ship (there was no curfew for officers). The quarter deck officer, a Lieutenant Junior Grade, seemed peeved and un-amused that we had had a killer night on the town while he had had to stand watch. We each saluted twice and retired to our staterooms. At 0800 hrs. I woke up to banging on my door, a dry mouth and a splitting headache.

"What?" Now *I* was peeved and un-amused.

"Doc, we need you on Level 4 on the double." A high pitched voice of a yeoman came through the door." Commander Starling is in serious pain."

Great. Instead of a beeper, late night surgery and fatigue, I had the mother of all hangovers, and the ship's Executive Officer was waiting for me to perform miracles. What a trade-off. Crawling out of my rack, stepping over the crumpled whites strewn on the deck in the order I had removed them only hours earlier, I struggled into my working khakis, and walked up two decks, slowly. A lieutenant was standing outside the X.O.'s door.

"He's waiting for you, Doc."

I tapped softly on the door, listened for the muffled "Come" and stepped into his stateroom. Perhaps "stateroom" is overstating the rectangular box that served as the X.O.'s sanctuary, but it certainly surpassed the spaces the rest of us had, if not in creature comforts, then in size.

Commander Starling was lying on his back, sweating, pale and in significant pain.

"Sir, what's the matter?"

"Doc, I hurt my back. It's killing me."

He wasn't kidding. I examined him carefully. He had excruciating pain in his low back, mid-lumbar region. No bruises or abrasions, and although he had no reflex in his left patella tendon, sensation was intact throughout both legs.

"Commander, how did this happen?"

Long silence.

"Doc, I fell. Hurt my back. Give me something."

I gave him 8 mg. of morphine intra-muscular, told him to rest and I'd be back. I needed more information and knew he wasn't about to give it to me. I closed the door behind me and noted the lieutenant who was studying the overhead as if looking for the answer to the question he knew was coming.

"What's the deal...?"

"Uh..." he continued to look any and everywhere, but at me.

"Lieutenant...?" I was emphatic.

"Doc, uh..." he lowered his brown eyes and looked directly at me. "This stays between me and you, right?"

I nodded.

"The X.O. got pretty boozed up last night at the Admiral's party. He walked out on the balcony, started to pee over the balustrade, lost his balance and did a one and a half gainer onto the ground. He landed smack on his butt." He stifled a laugh. "We had to carry him back to the ship."

"Well, guess what, Lieutenant. He's got a compression fracture of L-3, 4."

"Oh, Christ! Doc, you'd better tell the Admiral and Captain ASAP. They're waiting to see you topside. Good luck."

Good luck? What did that mean? I didn't cause this problem but it landed in my lap and I had to resolve it.

Fortunately, I had a set of clean Trop Whites since the uniform I had worn the previous night was the uniform I had woken up in—crumpled, with Sangria stains surrounded by salsa stains. My adrenaline was pumping and I made it up to the Captain's quarters. The Admiral, Captain and Operations Officer were sitting there, nary a smile in the crowd. The Admiral spoke first.

"What's your assessment, doctor?"

"Well, Sir, the X.O. has sustained a compression fracture of his lumbar spine resulting in loss of knee reflex and inability to ambulate. He may require surgical decompression."

Obviously, this was not something the top brass could easily sweep under the rug.

"What do you recommend?"

"Sir, I feel we must get him to the nearest U.S. Naval Hospital, ASAP."

The Admiral pondered for a moment, turned to the Captain and said, "Captain, set sail for Naples."

Christ. I felt like Helen of Troy, the face that launched a thousand ships. The whole 6th Fleet Task Force in Barcelona was leaving for Naples. The carrier, our cruiser, three tin cans (destroyers), a supply ship and an oiler—all based on my "assessment".

"Thank you, doctor. I'll expect your written report on the X.O. by tomorrow."

"Yes, Sir. Thank you, Sir," I responded, saluted and left.

After closing the door behind me, the Lieutenant approached and whispered, "Doc, the Admiral is *very* interested in your report."

Hmmm.

I returned to my stateroom and took "the-morning-after-the- night-before" shower—not a regular shower, a Navy shower. This entertaining indulgence lasts exactly 30 seconds—15 seconds to get wet and then turn off the water. You apply soap and shampoo while shivering. Then you have 15 seconds to wash off the soap and shampoo by which time the water is just getting warm before turning it off again. I completed the first 15 seconds, turned off the water and shampooed my hair. At that point, the alarm for general quarters went off.

All water is immediately shut down throughout the ship and all personnel must report to their stations. The Captain chose a hell of a time for a drill! I bolted out of the shower stall and whacked my shin on the vertical foot plate. I toweled off the soap as best I could, put on my khakis and cap with soap and water dribbling down the back of my neck and bumped into the Skipper (Captain) on the way to sick bay.

"Looks like you just came out of the shower, Doc."

No shit. "Yes, Sir, I did."

To this day I still take Navy showers, but I don't turn the water off to shampoo. Lynn even learned to take Navy showers, but she grew out of that real quick.

The next morning I wrote the following report: "Commander Starling suffered an accidental fall resulting in a compression fracture of the lumbar spine, possibly requiring surgery at nearest Naval hospital." So I told the truth and nothing but the truth, though maybe not the whole truth.

CHAPTER TWENTY SIX

CORFU: CUT TO CURE

*You need a little chaos in your soul to give
birth to a dancing star.*
Friedrich Wilhelm Nietzsche,
German philosopher

"Get Back",
The Beatles (1969)

We sailed the Mediterranean for six months, the Russians trailing us in a destroyer at a distance of several miles. Re-fueling at sea always took place at night, the oil tanker keeping a ten-knot pace with us, sixty feet to our starboard. The decks were softly lit by overhead, covered dull-red lights so no adversary air craft could spot us and knock out two ships at once. Heavy cables were established between our two ships and the ten inch oil fueling hose was then passed to our ship via the cables. The leading nose was a steel cone which fit into the cruiser's oil tank port and clamped securely in place. What a sight. Two enormous Navy ships traveling silently in the darkness, sixty feet apart, cutting through the water with double wakes, communicating to each other by hand signals or blinking lights, all in subdued red lighting which danced on the surface of the swiftly moving water.

I was actually getting paid to watch all this.

A sailor guided the steel conical nose into the oil tank receptacle but the momentum of our ship suddenly forced the hose off center, snipping off the sailor's four fingers at the middle joints. Blood and screams were everywhere. We carried him down to sick bay and placed him on the operating table. Two hours of revision amputation and lots of morphine followed. Since I wasn't a hand surgeon, we pulled into port the next day and transferred him to the huge Naval Hospital in Naples, Italy.

As I was returning to the pier, an incredible coincidence occurred. The aircraft carrier *USS Franklin D. Roosevelt (CV-42)* had tied up next to us and I bumped into one of the docs aboard, George Miller, a classmate of mine from medical school. We recognized each other instantly and chatted for a minute. He was carrying a medium sized cardboard box with what looked like smoke seeping out the sides. Actually it was dry ice, preserving remnants of brain tissue found in the helmet of an A-6 pilot who had flown off the carrier and later crashed into the ocean in the dark of night. True or not, the story I got from George was that the pilot and his navigator may have become complacent, possibly mesmerized by the exotic mixture of flying their jet at low level and high speed in the pitch black of night. Whatever else remained, the sharks had removed it by the time the USS *Franklin D. Roosevelt* located the crash site at dawn.

We received our mail by military helicopter twice a week. "Hey, German, you got one." This was a rare treat and I snatched the letter with excitement. It was from Carol and though we had now been separated for nearly two years, it was news from home in that beautiful handwriting of hers.

"Dear Rich—I know you want happiness for me as I do for you. I have met a wonderful man from California and we plan to marry as soon as you get back to the U.S. and sign the divorce papers. Can I count on your cooperation? Carol".

It was over.

Eight years and it's finally over. I felt many things— concern for Lynn and our relationship, finality, loss, change and yes, a bit of relief. Life goes on.

A week later we dropped anchor in deep water off the beautiful island of Corfu, Greece, since our ship was too long to tie up to the pier. In fact, only two ports in the Med had piers big enough for a ship of our size— Barcelona, Spain and Gaeta, Italy. I had been reading a book called "Z" which was about the coup that took over political power from King Constantine in 1967. At that time, this book had been banned in Greece. Of course, it intrigued the Greek yachtsmen I had met at the Corfu Yacht Club. We did a trade: he got the book I had smuggled off the ship for him, and I got his 22-foot sailboat for the day.

Once again, navigation was not my strong suit, and not knowing the area I sailed over to what I thought was an island, and then returned after a four hour sail. The Greek started screaming at me from the dock, "You idiot, you idiot!" Seems the "island" was actually Albania, one of the five communist countries (China, North Korea, North Viet Nam and Cuba) off limits to all military personnel. The boat and I could have been seized. Obviously, he was not worried about me. I now had the dubious distinction of having sailed into restricted waters of two countries off limits to military personnel!

The next day was a beautiful Sunday. I was about to leave for shore when the loudspeaker squawked an emergency call.

"Lieutenant German. Report to sick bay immediately. Repeat. Report to sick bay immediately."

A sailor had fallen ten feet off a ladder onto the steel deck. He had been transported to sick bay and the medical corpsman was taking his blood pressure.

"Doc, it hurts like shit. Right here."

He put his hand over his upper abdomen, just below his left rib cage.

He had a large red contusion over his left rib cage margin, a tender silent abdomen, blood pressure 80/40 and a pulse of 130. Diagnosis: ruptured spleen, a surgical emergency. I started an IV of normal saline and ran it full blast. The ship did not have the equipment for this type of major surgery so we piled him onto the liberty launch and took him to shore. Fortunately, it was a calm day and the boat ran smoothly at a fast clip. We carried him off the boat on a stretcher and laid him on the dock. There was no ambulance available so we stopped a truck, loaded him onto the flatbed and raced to the local hospital. Unfortunately, the road was not so smooth and he winced at every bump, a sign of generalized peritonitis, an inflammation of the peritoneal lining of the abdominal cavity which causes pain. I had learned this valuable sign as an intern when evaluating a patient for possible early appendicitis. My resident at the time asked the patient to stand up on his toes and come down hard on his heels. The patient had winced and placed his hand on his right lower abdomen, right over the appendix. Revised diagnosis—acute appendicitis, with localized peritonitis. The medical dictum: listen (observe) carefully and the patient will give you his diagnosis.

I felt as though I were in a M.A.S.H. unit. Holding a bottle of saline over my injured sailor, I sat on a box in the back of a flat bed truck, bouncing our way to the hospital on a hot, humid June day amidst drop-dead gorgeous scenery. The hospital was small and modest—no air conditioning, but adequate, with a responsive staff. Key personnel had been notified. The hospital surgeon, Greek of course, was pleasant. We conversed in limited English, and some French which I had taken in prep school and college. He offered to let me do the surgery, and I didn't object. We drew blood for type and cross, removed his clothes, shaved his abdomen with warm soapy water and a razor, hung a bottle of blood and shot over to the OR. We quickly scrubbed up. Bare-chested and wearing only white scrub pants, and white surgical caps, we entered the OR. The nurse helped me into the gown, but the sleeves were too short for me. The nurse covered the gap between my sleeves and gloves with two rags around my wrists—a major breach in sterile protocol—-but my patient was bleeding to death, and I would have operated with bare hands if necessary.

"Knife, please."

The scrub nurse did not speak English but she certainly understood the universal language of surgical hand signals. She placed the knife in my extended right hand.

I made a 6-inch long oblique incision just below the left rib cage (subcostal incision) and blitzed through the subcutaneous fat, deep fascia and muscle in very rapid succession. His blood pressure was low, 80/60 with a rapid pulse, so there was not much bleeding from my incision through the abdominal wall. What bleeding there was could be adequately controlled by placing a sterile lap towel over the wound edges and proceeding to the more important, life-threatening bleeding inside his belly.

In dire, near death surgical emergencies I have made the incision without general anesthesia and without scrubbing up, wearing only gloves and short sleeve scrubs (no time to scrub, no time to put on a gown). It becomes very messy—you do what you have to do, and in those cases it's usually not enough. If by some miracle the patient stabilizes on the table and starts to respond to pain, the anesthesiologist will then administer appropriate anesthesia. If by some miracle the patient survives, chances are he is not going to die from exposure to my non-sterile bare forearms fishing around in his belly to save his life.

I pointed to the now nearly empty pint of blood hanging on the IV pole, then gestured emphatically with two fingers. Translation—"Get two more units of blood, NOW!"

We popped through the delicate peritoneal lining and into the abdominal cavity. It was filled with almost 2 liters of dark venous blood. All I could see were lakes of blood interspersed among loops of bowel. The rest of the organs were "under water". I reached blindly into the left upper quadrant. Blood was up to my forearms and completely obscured my vision. I felt for the spleen. My fingers coursed along the smooth surface and suddenly dove into a huge crevice.

The spleen had been torn in half. I pushed several large OR towels into the splenic bed and compressed the spleen with my right hand to control the bleeding. We gave more blood and vigorously suctioned the pooled blood from the abdomen. As the level of blood receded, other abdominal organs came into view—the right lobe of the liver, omentum, transverse colon, ascending colon, small bowel mesentery, left lobe of the liver and finally my right hand holding a bunch of blood soaked towels against the spleen.   Still keeping my right hand compressing the spleen, we irrigated the entire abdomen with liters of sterile saline to remove all blood and clots. No further bleeding and no other injuries. Thank God! By this time more blood had been given and the patient was stabilizing hemodynamically. BP 130/82, pulse down to 100.

This was the moment for everyone to take a deep breath, regroup and get ready for the next step. All instruments to remove the spleen were placed on the Mayo stand: 2 long (14 inch) curved Kelly clamps, O and 2-O long silk ties, long curved Metzenbaum scissors, 3-O silk suture ligatures, a long curved Deaver retractor.

With my right hand still compressing the spleen, I reached in with my left hand and pinched the vascular pedicle (blood supply) between my index and middle finger. I slowly removed the towels with my right hand. I could feel that damned splenic artery pulsating between my pinched fingers, daring me to release my grip, in which case all hell would break loose. The blood saturated towels were removed one after the other until we could see the deep fracture of the spleen. I grasped the long curved Kelly and placed it across the rich vascular pedicle (the stalk that provides the artery and vein to an organ) supplying the spleen, dancing between the delicate tail of the pancreas beneath and the easy- to-tear splenic vein above, dancing between the devil and the deep blue sea.

Slowly I compressed the clamp, hearing it ratchet down until it had occluded the pedicle. Silence. Irrigate.

No bleeding. I could feel my heart pounding. This was the critical moment. I applied a second Kelly clamp just distal (behind and closer to the spleen) to the first and divided the pedicle between the two clamps with the long scissors. No bleeding. The proximal clamp was gently dancing to the tune of the arterial pulse. I handed the clamp handle to my Greek assistant and carefully, very carefully, tied off the pedicle with a double throw surgeon's square knot. I removed the clamp. No bleeding. I irrigated with saline. No bleeding. My heart rate was coming down. I placed a second 2-O silk reinforcing tie proximally, tied off the distal clamp with an O silk tie and divided the ligaments holding the spleen to the diaphragm and left kidney. No bleeding. I removed the spleen. It was nearly fractured in two. It stared back at me, devil that it was. I put it in a pan and the nurse handed it off the table. Good riddance! I became aware of the sweat trickling down my neck and back. Let's finish this damn case.

The patient had survived.

I had nearly died!

CHAPTER TWENTY SEVEN

GOING HOME

Carpe diem. (Seize the day!)
Horace, Roman poet

"Tie a Yellow Ribbon 'Round the
Old Oak Tree...",
Tony Orlando, 1973

I was lying on my bunk catching up on some reading. There was a knock on my cabin door. "The Captain wants to see you, Lieutenant."

Now what? This doesn't happen very often. With a degree of anxiety I climbed six flights of nearly vertical metal stairs two steps at a time and tapped on the Captain's door. It was partially opened.

"Come on in, Doc." He had a pleasant, non-threatening expression on his face. That was a relief. "Your year on the *Albany* is nearly up. I need to fill out your transfer orders for your second year. Do you have any preferences?"

Wow! The Navy always calls the shots. What gives? But here was my chance.

"If I have any choice, Sir, it would be California."

"How does Long Beach Naval Hospital sound?"

"It sounds perfect, Sir. Thank you, Sir".

"Be packed and ready to go by 1000 hrs. tomorrow. A helicopter will pick you up and take you to the carrier *USS Roosevelt*. You'll be flown off the carrier to the Naval Air

Station in Naples, Italy and then home to McGuire Air Force Base in New Jersey. Good luck." He smiled and handed me my orders.

"Yes, sir and thank you, Sir!"

"And by the way, Doc," he continued, "your medical report on the X.O. last month was much appreciated. We'll miss you."

So there it was—pay back for a report that spared the brass embarrassment. Love it! My heart was pounding and singing for joy. What incredible luck. Lynn and I will both be in California—yeah!!

I had bought my British racing green TR-6 convertible for $2,000 when we docked in Naples the month before, and had it shipped to New York. My adrenaline was over the top—I was going home!!

The next morning at 1000 hrs. I stood on the aft deck of the *Albany* in my Service Dress Khakis carrying my fully packed Marine duffle bag that contained all of my worldly goods. Two TALOS missiles were resting on the launcher so the helicopter was unable to land on deck. It hovered 200 feet above the aft end of the ship as we were cutting through the Med at about 10 knots, the helicopter keeping pace with the ship. It was a dramatic moment. The cable was lowered and the harness placed over my head and under my arms.

"Request permission to depart the ship, Sir."

"Permission granted, Lieutenant."

A salute to the flag and damned if they didn't whistle me off: "Lieutenant, U.S. Navy, departing". The helicopter blades were pounding and I felt the powerful pull of the harness as my feet lifted off the steel deck for the last time.

I hung from the cable for several minutes as the hydraulic lift slowly hoisted me up and the helicopter banked steeply away. The *Albany,* my home for a year, disappeared in the distance like a small speck on the ocean.

Thirty minutes later we approached the carrier. The Navy A-4 Skyhawks and A-6 Intruders were practicing cat-shots (launches) and touch-and-go landings, so we hovered off the starboard side of the ship. If only I had had a camera. One jet nearly had a ramp strike (into the aft end of the carrier), went to MRT (maximum rated thrust) on his TF-30-P6 engine, and barely missed crashing into the ocean, his left wing coming within 20 feet of the water. He circled around and in a trembling voice asked permission for another attempt to land on the carrier. We were monitoring all aircraft-to-ship communications on our headsets and heard the Air Boss deny permission. The pilot was bingo'ed to Naples 35 minutes away, a much safer option considering his mental state after nearly killing himself.

After we had landed on the *Roosevelt,* the flight deck officer approached me. "Doc, I don't know what connections you have but we have orders to fly you out right away. Follow me and keep your head down." He led me to a twin engine turbo-prop C-2 aircraft with eight seats. I stowed my duffle bag, buckled my shoulder and seat harnesses, and looked across the carrier deck through a small window. The engines went to full throttle and the catapult shot us down the track, thrusting me back into my seat. As the wheels left the ship the aircraft dropped to about 40 feet above the water. Slowly we regained altitude and headed for Naples. What an E-ticket ride!

Another benefit of my "downplayed" report on the X.O. was a two week pass in Europe prior to my deployment back to the States. I flew to Copenhagen and bicycled around town. To this day I have never tasted a more delicious ice cream cone than the one I had in Tivoli Gardens. After a short boat ride over to Malmo, Sweden for the day, I was off to West Berlin on a military flight.

After changing into my civilian clothes, with military I.D. and passport in my pocket, I headed toward Checkpoint Charlie, the dividing line between Communist East Berlin and Allied West Berlin. The fifty-foot walk from West Berlin to East Berlin was sobering: as the red- and white-striped pedestrian barrier lifted to let me pass, I left the safety of West Berlin and walked beneath the conning towers at the other end, manned with the usual Communist overkill—two guards and two machine guns.

West Berlin was free, bustling and colorful; East Berlin, in stark contrast, was subdued, depressing and gray. Remnants of World War II were ubiquitous—the façade of a cathedral was pockmarked with bullet holes and the entire interior had been gutted and was filled with rubble. One structure after another repeated this pattern. People shuffled about with no expressions on their faces. Communism had taken its toll and economic deprivation was painfully obvious. By chance, I bumped into a fellow officer who was in uniform. After a few minutes of conversation he expressed concern that I was not in uniform. He was certain that the Geneva Convention dictated that any active duty military personnel be in uniform, for identification purposes, at all times when entering a Communist country. By that definition, I had inadvertently had become a spy! He convinced me that I should either discard my military I.D., or hide it in my shoe and pray.

Fortunately, I had obtained my passport prior to entering the service, so it showed no indication of my current military status. As I approached Checkpoint Charlie, my heart pounded. All visitors exiting East Berlin were required to enter a trailer guarded by armed East German soldiers, one at the entrance and one at the exit. I slipped my passport into a slot in the wall and saw it disappear. Heart rate 130. Silence. Finally, my passport reappeared through the slot and the East German soldier handed it to me and pointed to the exit. Heart rate 140. As I left the trailer, I walked past the conning tower with my eye on that red and white crossbar. I showed my passport to the American M.P. and walked on through to freedom. Heart rate 80. What a jerk I had been! So now I had tempted fate three times: sailing in Cuban and Albanian waters, and strolling through East Berlin as a "spy". Time to go home.

CHAPTER TWENTY EIGHT

CALIFORNIA DREAMIN'

"Two roads diverged in a wood, and I—
I took the one less traveled by,
and that has made all the difference."
Robert Frost, poet

"All the leaves are brown,
and the sky is gray . . ."
"California Dreamin' ", The Mamas and Papas
(1966)

August 1970. I landed at McGuire Air Force Base and my parents met me—a poignant moment, as Dad had been a Navy Lieutenant during World War II. Mom hugged me and cried, Dad gave me a salute and a big hug. What a feeling—I was back on terra firma, U.S.A. I picked up my TR-6 in Bayonne, N.J., spent the night in Madison, Connecticut with my folks and then headed to Boston to see Lynn. She was eight and such a grown-up, beautiful young girl. She was waiting on the lawn. She didn't recognize the car but when I got out she ran to me, leaped into my arms and held on for minutes in silence— both of us with tears streaming down our cheeks. A beautiful moment and one I will never forget.

"Well, Lynn, we're all going to be in California soon."

"I know, Dad, let's sing our song." And there we were, Lynn and I sitting on the lawn singing "California Dreamin' ".

The Navy gave me ten days before I had to report to Long Beach Naval Hospital. I spent a few happy days with friends and family in Connecticut, packed up my shiny new TR-6, including a care package stuffed with home-made goodies from Oma, and headed out across the country on Route 66. I was so excited about getting to California that I drove non-stop from Connecticut to St. Louis in 36 hours, crashed for 4 hours and then drove to Tulsa, Oklahoma. After a good night's sleep I drove to Tempe, Arizona and spent the evening with a friend from college.

It was August, hotter than hell, dry, dull and devoid of an ocean. On to California. I arrived at Terminal Island, Long Beach Naval Air Station at midnight. I presented my transfer papers to the Marine guard at the entrance gate and he reviewed them in silence for a moment. He handed the papers back to me, snapped a sharp salute without saying a word and I drove to the BOQ (Bachelor Officers' Quarters) and went up to my assigned room on the third floor. I shared a common bathroom with a Navy pilot recently returned from Nam, but we each had our own room. It felt good to be in California and a Navy officer to boot.

The next morning I got up early and drove north on the Long Beach Freeway to the 405 Freeway south and north again on the 605 Freeway to the Carson Street exit and Long Beach Naval Hospital, my home for the next year. Orientation took most of the day but I was dying to see the OR. Well, I got my chance. The senior surgeon and Chief of Surgery, Capt. Roger Hart, paged me.

"German, I've got a hot gall bag. I need you to assist me."

Hot damn! I went to the surgical locker room and changed into my scrubs.

I thought to myself, "I've been transplanted to heaven!"

The case was underway and I walked up to the OR table, arms dripping wet from the soapy scrub. The male scrub nurse welcomed me, introduced me around, and gowned and gloved me. What a tingle! To add icing to the cake, one of the techs turned the radio on at the request of the surgeon. *"Suite: Judy Blue Eyes"* by Crosby, Stills & Nash was playing. Here I was, at last in California, scrubbed in on a great case, all the natives were friendly and that haunting, transcending melody playing in the background. Like Dorothy's words in the *Wizard of Oz*, "We're not in Kansas (Rochester) anymore." Yes, indeed!

Capt. Hart took the knife and made a rapid 4-inch oblique incision, just below and parallel to the right costal margin—down through the dermis, sub-cutaneous fat and Scarpa's fascia all in one motion.

"It's getting to the point where I'm no fun anymore ... I am sorry".

"Rich, cauterize those bleeders. Keep up with me."

"Yes, Captain", I responded.

"Rich, no military talk in the OR. I'm Roger, you're Rich. O.K.?"

"O.K."

Like catching a California wave out surfing, I felt ahead of the curve. I was an intrinsic part of the operation and felt the thrill of being in the thick of things. He was depending upon me, and I sure as hell was not going to disappoint him. His blade sliced through the fascia, exposing the rich, dark red muscle belly of the rectus abdominus, and in a flash popped through the peritoneum.

"I am yours, you are mine, you are what you are...and you make it hard"

No more somber silence and pervasive paranoia of being a pyramid program surgical resident in the University OR. This was life. Real life. Exhilarating life. I was surgically surfing my way to becoming a skilled professional. I stoically held the thrill of the moment to myself which only intensified the excitement.

"Chestnut brown canary, ruby throated sparrow, sing the song,

don't be long, thrill me to the marrow..."

I was home. Home in California, home in the vibrancy, home in the belly!

"Do do do do do,   do do do do do do,   do do do do do,   do do do do"

By this point in my training, I was 100% dedicated to a future surgical career and got into the OR at every opportunity, primarily at the invitation of a fully trained surgeon doing his time in the service as well. Capt. Hart was full-time Navy and equally cooperative in getting me into my size 8 surgical gloves to assist him. To this day, he performed the absolute, hands-down, fastest cholecystectomy (gall bladder removal) I have ever seen—17 minutes, skin-to-skin (from incision to dressing).

The hospital was a four story, acute care facility for active and retired military personnel and their families.

Most of our surgical cases were of an elective nature, although we did take care of some injured sailors and Marines sent to us from Viet Nam, via Guam. One Marine needed shrapnel to be removed from his leg. He had been injured in an explosion, separated from his unit and eventually captured by the Viet Cong. Incredibly, he escaped in the middle of the night and floated down the Mekong Delta where he was able to send out an S.O.S. A Huey H-1 rescue helicopter responded and plucked him from the jungle by dropping down a cable. Once he had been hoisted aboard, he was given a parachute and thanked his guardian angel for his rescue. At that moment, a SAM (surface to air missile) slammed into the helicopter and split it in half, killing the pilot and co-pilot. The Marine jumped forward out of the remaining half of the helicopter and parachuted to safety. He spent two more days in the jungle, avoiding recapture and was eventually rescued by ground troops. I have cared for many military individuals who had faced far less trauma but carried permanent emotional scars. This Marine treated his experience like it was a walk in the park, and he insisted that I remove the shrapnel under local anesthesia. He was afraid a general anesthesia might kill him!

The Navy was good for me. I felt secure, appreciated, unpressured—and I played a lot of tennis. What a sensation to drive over to the Navy base courts on a sunny, warm February day, looking east to the snow laden San Bernardino mountains and thinking back to my frozen-tundra February days in Rochester. What a change! At any given intersection, I would see an old woody carrying a couple of surfers and their boards, a Porsche with a full ski rack and a blonde headed for the slopes, a convertible loaded with "Beach Betties" and me in my green TR-6, loving life.

My tennis partner, Crane, had just left Harbor General Hospital/UCLA as Chief Resident in Surgery, having opted for a full Berry Plan deferment before completing his two year military obligation. Luckily Viet Nam was starting to wind down so he had been assigned to Long Beach Naval Hospital. He taught me many valuable lessons in surgical techniques— how to one hand tie square knots, cut sutures on an angle to avoid cutting the knot, and cut only with the scissors tips to avoid cutting anything else inadvertently. I perfected bowel anastomosis (connecting the two ends of the resected bowel by suturing technique) and would always reinforce "the angle of sorrow", that vulnerable part of the bowel closure which would invariably leak unless great care was taken with the sutures. These were some of the "pearls" I learned under his tutelage and it was a fun partnership in and out of the OR, on and off the courts. I started making tough decisions and learned how to anticipate and avoid complications. I also learned that "pearl droplets" showing through a patient's hospital gown were an early sign of impending wound infection—remove the sutures, probe the wound with a sterile q-tip and search for that deep lying silent wound abscess. Once again, the mantra of observe, observe, observe and think prevailed. Long days in the OR were balanced by long weekends sailing over to Catalina Island. I knew I was now a Californian, not just a transplanted Connecticut Yankee.

My last few months in the Navy were running out, and the reality of continuing my surgical training became paramount. Although these last two years had counted for nothing in the way of formal surgical training, I had a wealth of experience that I knew would put me in good stead and ahead of the rest of the pack. As luck would have it, Crane arranged for an interview with the Director of the

Surgical Residency Program at Harbor General Hospital/UCLA Medical Center on Friday. Three days later, on Monday, I received a call from the secretary.

"Dr. German, you've been accepted to our second year residency program in surgery. Congratulations".

Pinch me! Pinch me!

Lynn, Carol and her new husband were now in Los Altos Hills, south of San Francisco. A quick flight to Los Angeles meant frequent visits with Lynn, and life had started again.

So there we were, Lynn and I with our feet in the warm Southern California sand watching the sunset, and once again we sang our song:

> *"All the leaves are brown and the sky is gray*
> *I've been for a walk on a winter's day*
> *I'd be safe and warm if I was in L.A.*
> *California Dreamin' on such a winter's day"*

Like it or not, I was pretty much a "Disneyland Dad". I only saw Lynn every couple of week-ends when she would fly down on PSA (Pacific Southwest Airlines), SFO to LAX. But better than Disneyland was Knott's Berry Farm, and better than KBF was the Pike in Long Beach. The Pike was a Saturday staple, a huge amusement park right on the beach replete with the fat lady, bearded lady, snake charmer, carnie hawker, white and pink cotton candy on a stick, hot dogs with an open tub of Gulden's mustard always buzzing with flies, and cold cokes in the bottle. But our absolute favorite was the Wild Mouse Ride which to this day amazes me that it somehow escaped major catastrophe. We sat in the tiny 2 seat cart which ran on 4 wheels over 2 rails high up in the air, made sudden 90 degree turns and abrupt drops, and to my knowledge never followed a well established law of physics which otherwise dictated that the entire car should lift off the rails and catapult into outer space, or make a 300 foot flight over the entire park and into the Pacific Ocean. I'm not a perfect man, but God was our co-pilot and would always guide us back to safety and, by comparison, a boring ride on the Thunderbolt roller-coaster.

When it was not my week-end to be dad, I would walk 3 blocks from tiny apartment down to the beach and play some solo Frisbee. I had it down to an art, throwing the Wham-O from water's edge out over the ocean at a 45 degree angle where the on-shore breeze would always carry it high in the air and back over the beach, all while I darted back and forth in the sand to capture the disc in mid-air as it came zooming back. Most of the time I was able to catch it. One time I didn't. The wind caught it and sent it flying high on the beach where it nearly decapitated a young woman, strawberry blond, marble blue-green eyes and drop dead gorgeous, sitting on a towel in khaki shorts and a blue tank top.

"Gosh, I'm sorry, I'm so sorry", I said gasping for air as I ran to retrieve my Frisbee.

"Oh, that's O.K. But wouldn't it be easier if you had a partner?" she oh-so subtly inquired.

"Why yes, of course. By the way, I'm Rich."

"And I'm Christine."

~

The End

EPILOGUE

This book covers the first eight years of my training as a surgeon, from the start of medical school in September 1963 through my internship and first year surgical residency, followed by two years in the Navy, ending in 1971.

The rigors of medical school are very real, competition ever present, but the energy needed to get through the varied courses in a four-year liberal arts college can now be focused on one single overriding objective—understanding the structure and function of the human body in health and disease. This relatively narrow focus is a great advantage for learning, especially since the entire four-year medical curriculum is inter-related, and therefore the knowledge gained is additive. The ultimate goal is the ability to correctly diagnose disease processes and choose the appropriate treatment.

Each year of surgical training lends itself to a geometric progression of technical skills and accountability. There is just too much to learn, and absorbing the prodigious amount of information does not allow the relatively leisure approach to information that one was afforded in college. Each successive step is a greater stretch than the previous one.

I did not understand this as a first year med student, let alone a junior in college which, more or less, is when this book starts out. I was carried through my first three years of med school like a cork on the ocean, reliant on my environment (professors, anatomy lab, exams) to direct my energy. My experience in Newfoundland changed all that. I became proactive toward my future and it was that catalyst that focused my determination to spend the rest of my professional life as a surgeon. Fourth year med school was a formality, albeit a significant learning experience, a necessary transition on my way to graduation and internship where I met "God", my omnipotent, omniscient and omnipresent Chief Resident who wielded power over life and death as a house officer.

My last years in Rochester, spent as a first year surgical resident in 1969, represented a paradigm shift in my life—marital separation, leaving a surgical program after six years and joining the U.S. Navy during an imposing military conflict (Viet Nam). That was both the nadir of my life, as well as the catapult to great opportunities which played themselves out during my Navy experience.

Once I arrived back on United States soil, namely California, my future opened up and I was given the chance to pursue my dream.

The principles and lessons that I learned during these first eight years of my medical training have been equally applicable to the many challenges that I have faced throughout my life, whether social, personal, professional or financial. At the low point of those eight years, it was my decision to face personal responsibility for my circumstances which became the catalyst for success. Determination and stamina, which are necessary ingredients to confronting what appear at the time to be insurmountable obstacles, provided the means for overcoming those challenges and experiencing the satisfaction and joy of personal achievement. For me, medicine has been a wonderful discipline and I feel rewarded to have had the opportunity to say, "I have saved a life".

There have been a great many technical advances since my days as a student and resident, and they have revolutionized the approach to and outcome of many diseases. Hodgkins' Disease now can be cured in most cases and my friend Binky could have survived instead of dying at age 16. Spectacular gains have been made in treating certain cancers via chemotherapeutic agents and radiotherapy. Endoscopic techniques play a major role in vascular, orthopedic, thoracic, general and gynecologic surgery, and both post-operative pain and hospital stay have been greatly reduced. Transplantation surgery has gone from its embryonic stages when I was a med student to spectacular achievements that occur on a daily basis today. And who could have conceived of robotic surgery, which gives the surgeon the ability to do extremely precise procedures from a distant location?

Of course, with every new technologic advance comes greater specialization to insure absolute competence among the physician in his or her field of expertise. My experience in a small hospital on a tiny island off the north coast of Newfoundland during the summer before my final year in med school was a pivotal point in my career. It was an opportunity to evaluate and treat patients almost entirely on my own, to apply all I had learned to this point in my education about the emotional, humanistic, intellectual and technical aspects of medical care. This experience cemented my determination to become a surgeon, and it gave me confidence in my ability to think and act independently.

In addition to the different techniques to master and the expansion of medical knowledge, another factor that has changed in a surgeon's training over the last decades is the limitation of the work week to 80 hours. This development is the result of a tragic case in New York in 1986.

The death of a patient was related to sleep deprivation of a surgical resident. It is now mandated that a house staff intern or resident may not work over 80 hours in a seven day period, and woe be to the teaching hospital that violates this rule. Ironically, given the compulsive, driven nature of a surgeon, most residents prefer working longer hours to maximize their exposure to cases and the continuity of care. As a practicing solo surgeon, I was on call for my patients 24/7. A resident, on the other hand, is forced to sign out to another resident and may return the next morning to find that his patient went through a crisis that had to be resolved without his knowledge.

Like so many mandated changes to a system as complex as surgical resident training, this rule change certainly has had unintended consequences. The residents and attending staff surgeons alike are not soothed. The residents want maximum exposure, and the teaching staff dislikes the disruption in continuity of training and care based on artificial time constraints. The bottom line is that multiple studies of this mandated hourly work statute have not substantiated statistically significant improvement in patient care, morbidity or mortality. Nevertheless, the rule stands. The other side of the coin is the not unreasonable conclusion that residents tend to learn more while awake!

The reader may find it strange that I spent two years serving in the Navy, time that was taken out of my residency and did not contribute to my formal surgical training. It was 1969 and we were immersed in Viet Nam. Surgeons of all types, partially or fully trained, were desperately needed. And the vast majority of all doctors faced mandatory recruitment. Under the Berry Plan, doctors in training could choose the timing of their two-year military obligation in return for a guarantee that the government would honor that commitment and not yank them out of training in the middle of the academic year. This would have been disastrous since the resident would lose credit for that year in addition to time spent working for the military. Since the academic year for all internship and residency programs is from July 1 through the following June 30, being recruited and released from the military in any month other than June meant potential loss of credit for that academic year and a huge delay in formal training. I don't know of any physician who ran to Canada, burned his draft card or retained an attorney. Military service was just expected of a doctor during war time, and, more to the point, there was just too much to lose fighting the system. I for one found the military a convenient break that provided me with many rich and rewarding experiences, and I am proud to have had the chance to serve my country.

In my thirty–five year career as a practicing surgeon, I performed general, trauma, vascular and cancer surgery. Then another opportunity of a lifetime came my way: I was invited to be a visiting volunteer senior surgeon at Landstuhl Regional Medical Center in Germany, which receives all U.S. military injuries from Iraq and Afghanistan. It is the largest U.S. military hospital outside the continental U.S. In September, 2007 I helped perform surgery on the wounded warriors and once again came face to face with the powerful reality of war. I also came face to face with the incredible dedication and poignant human spirit of the American soldier, many having sustained horrific injuries. Having started my early surgical career in the Navy during Viet Nam, I came full circle and ended my surgical career by serving in yet another war. I returned to Landstuhl, Germany over Christmas week 2008 for another "tour of surgical duty", to immerse myself in that powerful and poignant environment which elevates appreciation for life and health to a higher order.

The path that a young man or woman must take to become a surgeon is a long and winding road. Success depends as much on total immersion in his or her work as it does upon the pursuit of intellectual honesty and integrity.

Finally, this book has been long in coming as I started it in 1970 while on the U.S.S. Albany CG-10, with very little to do for long periods of time. Through fits and starts, I have now completed it. If my experience is helpful to one patient, to one fellow doctor, to one human being facing his or her own personal challenges, than I am grateful. If not, at least my two daughters will have an insight into their Dad that perhaps they did not have before.